The Physiology of Eurythmy Therapy

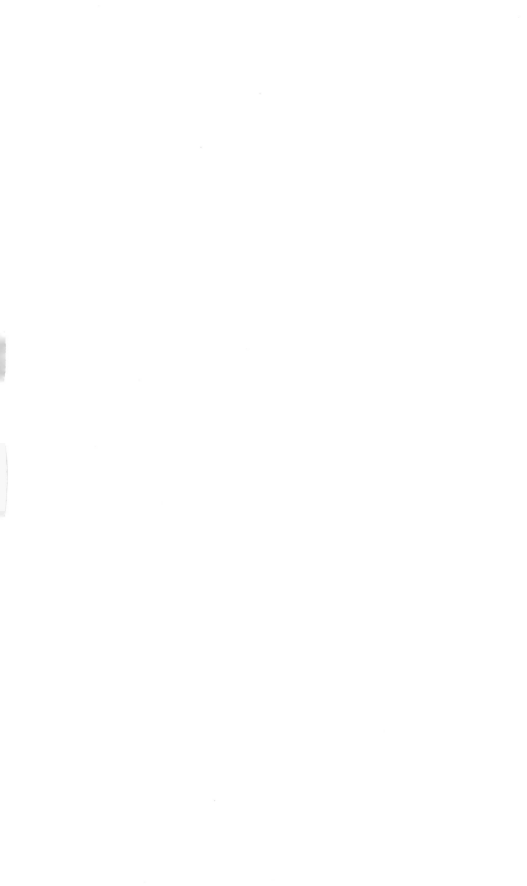

THE PHYSIOLOGY OF EURYTHMY THERAPY

Hans-Broder von Laue
Elke E von Laue

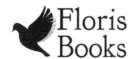

Floris Books

Translation from German by David Macgregor

First published in German as *Zur Physiologie der Heileurythmie*
in 2007 by Verlag am Goetheanum, Switzerland

English edition revised by the authors
First published in English by Floris Books in 2010
Third printing 2018

British Library CIP Data available
ISBN 978-086315-740-0
Printed by Lightning Source

Contents

Translator's Note on Pronunciation

The vowel sounds in the text follow German pronunciation. Equivalent English approximations are as follows:

A – as in 'ah' (bath)
E – as in 'eh' (bait)
I – as in 'ee' (beet)
O – as in 'oh' (boat)
U – as in 'oo' (boot)
Au – as in 'ow' (bout)
Ei – as in the personal pronoun 'I' (bite)

Ch – as in Scots 'loch,' not as in 'cheese'

1. Introduction

We dedicate this book to our friend Werner Barfod, a gifted eurythmist. What began as a friendship in our youth has grown into a sustained shared effort to grasp the anthroposophical foundations of eurythmy and medicine and make them fruitful in our own deeds. Questions and experiences to do with eurythmy therapy formed the bond. This is where our endeavours in eurythmy therapy meet the life's work of our friend: his struggle to find a spiritual understanding of the human being as a basis for eurythmy, so that it may remain capable of development.

This book has arisen over thirty years of working together: again and again the practice of eurythmy therapy met the theoretical scientific and medical striving to assess and systematize. On the one hand Steiner said that the 'empirical material' had been developed in the Eurythmy Therapy Course and that it was 'hardly necessary to go beyond what was given at that time' (p. 106). On the other hand, we have continually experienced how difficult it is to find common ground between the concerns of the physician and the practical ability of the eurythmy therapist.

Again and again we worked through the Eurythmy Therapy Course and the medical courses to track down the 'system of eurythmy therapy.' After all, Steiner said to the teachers, 'eurythmy therapy as a system was elaborated by me at the last medical course.'[1] The admonition of the adept, Isabella de Jaager, accompanied us just as vividly. She wrote in the prologue to the Eurythmy Therapy Course:

A living grasp of the human being and the world is a necessary
basis for its use. Only on this assumption will it [eurythmy
therapy] avoid becoming a system or something that is grasped and
applied in an abstract, intellectual way. (p. 136).

We present in this book the current state of our efforts, having presented and appraised the principles in several courses. We are well aware that certain correlations and conclusions will not be shared by all eurythmy therapists. Because the 'system of eurythmy therapy' implicit within the Eurythmy Therapy Course, is not explicitly elaborated, it is up to each therapist to seek their own 'system.' The ideas and experiences of one person may appear to another as 'invented and abstract.' In this respect what is put forward in this work should be taken as suggestion and hypothesis. Each may adopt into their own 'system' what fits their particular approach. If working in this way proves fruitful, that will be the proof of its validity.

Erna van Deventer-Wolfram, one of the two initiators of the Eurythmy Therapy Course, wrote in 1961

> In 1915 we young people had not the slightest idea why he gave
> this form for pedagogical practice, as we hardly understood any of
> the 'why' behind the whole teaching material of eurythmy. And, if
> we are honest, do we understand it any better today?

In all therapeutic endeavour, and with every illness, an individual approach and universal systematics need to be brought together afresh. Every single ill person has the right as an individual to be placed at the very centre of the therapeutic activity. They are at the same time entitled to know that the therapy for their illness can stand the scrutiny of critical scientific judgment. Neither the individual nor the universally scientific should be overvalued. This is valid in principle for all branches of medicine. Within anthroposophic medicine, the requirement to take into account what is individual in the ill person has a particular significance. In the case of eurythmy therapy, there is the danger that the individual path of healing of the particular patient may be overemphasized and that the systematic therapy for the illness withdraws into the background. This is probably connected to the fact that the 'system of eurythmy therapy' which was indicated by Steiner has not yet sufficiently been taken up by physicians and eurythmy therapists in a critical dialogue. The result of this is that the value of eurythmy therapy is far too little known among the public at large.

In this book we are proposing a systematization of the indications. The whole Eurythmy Therapy Course is based on the transformation of movement processes: how is the movement of speech transformed into eurythmy movement? This metamorphosis forms the initial point of departure for the arranging and organizing we are proposing. The therapeutic indications for the consonants which are mentioned in the Eurythmy Therapy Course provide the key: it is possible to discover a pattern, even if some of the pieces of the mosaic are not named. The mosaic can be completed if the whole composition has been harmoniously built up in one's own mind. The amplifications required bring some seekers to an experience of inner proof; for others the connections are no more than an arbitrary intellectual game. The harmonious arrangement of the whole series justifies our trust in its viability. Many of Rudolf Steiner's scattered indications can be better understood in the new context.

The indications for the vowels which we present here – including the additions of *Au* and *Ei* – are, on the other hand, only present in the text of the course up to a certain point. It may be obvious that language consists of the sounding together of vowels and consonants; yet it is still difficult to integrate this polarity into a therapeutic systematic arrangement. To do this it is necessary to make great leaps of thought. It would certainly be easier if clarifying 'hints' for the systematizing of therapeutic indications for the vowels were to be found. Such an outcome is unlikely. The only approach left, therefore, is to use our thinking and to create a holistic picture, from the few underpinning 'indications.' We present this now to eurythmy therapists and physicians to be tried, tested and developed. We hope there will be improvements and corroboration, objections and new therapeutic approaches and experiences. This work may lead to future studies into the efficacy of eurythmy therapy, and to clarify conceptually the therapeutic application of particular sequences of sounds.

This book could not have come about without the research work which we have undertaken over the course of many years at the Rüspe Study Centre and in Öschelbronn in Germany with Werner Barfod and Thomas Göbel, a research biologist. We owe much to this collaboration. We would also like to thank our medical and eurythmy therapy colleagues for their corrections and the suggestions which took us further on our path. We are particularly grateful to Angelika Jaschke, who has supported and encouraged our work over many years.

2. The Processes of the Etheric Body Between the Upper and Lower Human Being

Rudolf Steiner drew attention very early on to the possibility of a healing application for eurythmy. In the first course at Bottmingen a consonant sequence was mentioned, about which the following was said:

> If later on you are working with children or adults who are excited, restless and nervous, then this sequence of sounds *D–F–G–K–H* can produce a calming and relaxing effect. ... This group of sounds [*L–M–N–P–Q*] stimulates excitement. You have to let people do this who come into your lessons tired, exhausted and sleepy. Then they will become stimulated and interested.[1]

This first indication came about within a small circle. However, as early as 1913, in the introduction to the first eurythmy performance in Munich, Rudolf Steiner pointed to the three spheres of activity of the new art of movement: the manifestation of beauty in artistic eurythmy, the possibility of an educational application and, lastly, that 'we can also influence the human organism and soul-condition in a healthy way.'[2] Educational eurythmy was put into practice six years later in the first Waldorf school. Elisabeth Baumann and Erna Wolfram were led through their experiences at school and in public classes to ask about the metamorphosis of eurythmy into eurythmy therapy. The physicians who had been present in Munich originally had as yet been unable to take up the challenge of developing a new form of therapy. It was the eurythmists' will to heal and courage in asking, that in 1921 led to the Eurythmy Therapy Course.

The 1920 first medical lecture cycle, *Introducing Anthroposophical Medicine*, had for its theme 'the outer manifestation of the inner human being' in health and illness. A year later a double course took place: the second medical course, *Anthroposophical Spiritual Science and Medical Therapy*, in the mornings; and the Eurythmy Therapy Course (published as *Eurythmy Therapy* in English) in the afternoons. Both courses focus on the knowledge of an extended therapy. In the mornings the understanding of the human being necessary to establish the spiritual element of the therapeutic substance is described to the physicians. Steiner formulates the theme as a question: 'how can the different sheaths of the human being be influenced by substances outside the human being ... that can be used as remedies?'[3] It will be clear to the reader of both courses that for a holistic therapy it is necessary to understand the pole of substance with our cognitive forces, while eurythmy therapy forms the other pole within the spectrum of an extended therapy. In the former case the patient is passive – the medicines work largely without their participation – while in the latter healing has to be wished for and practised by the patient themselves. It must be achieved through independent practice.

The content of the Eurythmy Therapy Course was directed at the physicians. Steiner hoped that trained physicians would take up the therapeutic potential of eurythmy therapy and develop it further. But the impetus came from the impulse of the two therapists. Apart from the physicians, therefore, only eurythmists who had shown a definite therapeutic commitment were permitted to take part in the course. The course is basically addressed to the 'will to heal' of the eurythmists in order that a new therapeutic profession may be formed. Attention is drawn in the course to the shared task of physicians and eurythmy therapists: eurythmy therapy has a 'physiological aspect which has its seat in the spiritual' and this needs to be developed. The necessity of becoming aware of and developing the 'physiology of eurythmic activity' is emphasized on several occasions.

The aim of both courses is to get to know and learn to influence the life processes of the 'eurythmist's ether body' in health and illness. In both courses there is barely a mention of either a spiritual-karmic or a psychological background to pathology or therapy. The processes of the etheric body in illness and in health stand in the foreground. For an understanding of the human etheric body it is necessary to distinguish the workings of all four parts of the human being in the living processes.

In order to come to a picture of the physiological processes we may, as an introduction, draw on the lecture 'The Invisible Human Being Within Us.' This lecture provides a key to understanding the descriptions in the medical courses and in the Eurythmy Therapy Course. The multiplicity of processes which takes place simultaneously in the living body is differentiated into four levels. Each of these four categories is itself divided into a 'visible' and an 'invisible' part (Figure 1).

The 'visible' and the 'invisible' human being should be understood separately in the living processes, even though both aspects permeate each other on all four levels.

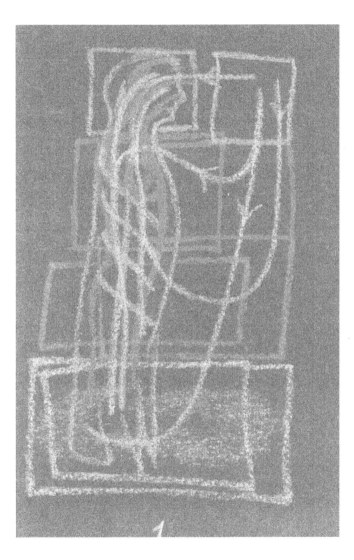

building up and
breaking down
processes in

the nervous and
sensory system

the respiratory
system

the circulatory
system

the metabolism
and limb system

Figure 1. The visible – invisible human being.
The functions of the upper and lower human being between the visible and
invisible human being. Based on Steiner's blackboard drawing in the lec-
ture, 'The Invisible Human Being Within Us' (CW 221, Feb 11, 1923).

On the visible side (the left side), the life processes are modified in that the 'visible astral body and the visible I' act directly on them. Catabolic (breaking down) processes are hereby brought into activity. The impulse for the catabolism of physiological potentials always arises from the higher parts of the human being acting directly. They appear in the soul as wakeful thinking, as dreaming feeling or as will. On the level of the etheric body, the processes are revealed as breaking down, catabolic physiological activities.

On the invisible side (right), the 'invisible I and astral body' bring about directly, in the ether body and the physical body, the building up processes which have to be transformed by the individual. The unconsciously working 'invisible I' shapes all the structures which arise anew in the human organism through this building up process. In the metabolism the building up processes work after the foreign nature of the nourishing substances has been overcome.

To this extent all living processes in the organism, both building up and breaking down are always permeated by the higher parts of the human being; they manifest in the ether body in fourfold fashion. Both the medical and the eurythmy courses we are considering here follow a similar presentation. When the working of the higher levels, the I and astral body, is spoken of in the lectures, Steiner hardly mentions soul-spiritual experiences but describes instead the effects in the ether body. Let us take an example to clarify the difference between soul experience and physiological processes. Grief is a soul-spiritual process which manifests visibly as weeping. The forming of tears out of the blood substance is the breaking down process activated in the ether body by grief. The experience of grief in the soul correlates with the living process of forming tears. It is the living processes that are focused on in these two courses, not the soul experience.

Let us summarize the polar processes in the ether body as the upper and lower human being. This describes not spatial differentiation but active qualities. The lower human being encompasses all processes in which building up takes place. building up has three tasks. First, after exertion, either the previous state of energy or the previous activity needs to be reconstituted (*maintaining*). Secondly, through *growth* the preconditions for enhanced abilities are brought about. Thirdly, *reproduction* leads to a complete renewal of the organism.

The higher sheaths – always with their 'visible' and 'invisible' components – shape these life processes. The individual steps of this building up activity can be observed. For instance one can measure the build-up of potential in a nerve, the phosphorylation or activation of a receptor or the synthesis of a new substance. In this way many individual steps can be examined in detail; however the overall purpose which builds up human function eludes such an approach. building up processes never appear in isolation. They are accompanied by formative, 'higher' activities which continually monitor, giving feedback and limiting 'lower' processes of building up activity.

The upper processes are determined through the direct intervention of the I and astral body; they shape the living processes. They include all those activities which have a catabolic character, breaking substance down. All perceptual functions belong here: the blood sugar level has to be monitored and regulated; the acidity of the blood; the degree of distension of the heart as it fills is monitored within the organism. In a mature organism, the upper processes appear as a depolarization (the lowering in the electrical potential) of a nerve, as the onset of a hormonal secretion or as the movement of a muscle. Even the combustion of an energy-rich substance in metabolism belongs physiologically to the activity of the upper human being. Table 1 overleaf describes as indications the processes of the upper and lower human being.

During the embryonic period all the steps of differentiation are initiated through the higher processes. The upper processes start and delimit new steps in development, they guide growth from the rudimentary starting tissue to the functional form of the organs; they drive development forward through selective growth inhibition (apoptosis), through the secretion of hormonlike messenger substances and by activating tiny little movements inside the differentiating tissue.

In Steiner's lectures, the upper and lower human being appear under very different names. In the first medical course we find:

You can only understand the polarity in the human being itself, when you know ... that the human being is put together as a duality so that it perceives its lower element from the vantage point of its higher ... Until you distinguish between this higher and lower, which is mediated through the heart, you will not be able to understand the human being, for there is a fundamental distinction between everything taking place in the lower activity of the organization and in the higher.[4]

In the first instance, Steiner used the word 'neurasthenic' for a preponderance of the upper human being; he called the opposite state 'hysteric.' These terms are not used again in subsequent lectures – they are too strongly associated with psychopathological concepts and not with living processes. These centres of forces are later called the 'upper human being' and the 'lower human being.'

The description refers to the processes in the ether body. The names 'upper' or 'lower' human being could easily give rise to misleading

Processes of the Ether Body

The upper human being	The lower human being
During organ development	
The cosmic soul and the I-organization guide the ether body to form the organs until they are mature enough to function Forming of cellular and extra-cellular components of organs Controlling the combining of soma, vessels, connective tissue and components of nerves Apoptosis	The cosmic soul and the I-organization guide the ether body in its growth until functional maturity Building up the potential for differentiation of rudimentary organs and functioning organs and of the extra-cellular matrix Building up the force of movement for the combining of soma, connective tissue and nerves
During organ usage	
Perception and guidance of inner processes on all levels: In the *nerve-sense system*: breaking down of nerve potentials, with tendency to hardening, mineralization, salt formation In the *rhythmic system*: induction of catabolic components of rhythms, preponderance of inhalation, acceleration of rhythmic processes In the *metabolic-limb system*: breaking down foreign nutritional substances, processes of combustion breaking down processes in the process of healing	Processes of conversion and building up which enable future effort: In the *nerve-sense system*: building up of nerve potentials, of nerve metabolism In the *rhythmic system*: induction of anabolic components of rhythms, preponderance of exhalation, deceleration of rhythmic processes In the *metabolic-limb system*: building up of individualized substance as general potential and for organ-specific activity, dissolution of 'old' individualized tissue building up processes in the process of healing
Further names and functions	
Arsenizing Formation of wedge shapes Hardening, calcification of tissues Mineralization Differentiating, steering Shaping force (*plastizierende Kraft*) Becoming wilful organically Using existing substances	Albumenizing Maceration, softening Dissolution of individualized tissue Pulverizing Jumbling up, bringing into chaos Welling force (*plastische Kraft*) Becoming selfless organically Forming substances anew

Table 1.

spatial attributions. Both forces work together simultaneously in the head and in the metabolism. The quality of the activity in question is the decisive factor, not the location. It is stated in the Eurythmy Therapy Course:

> When eurythmy is used for therapeutic purposes it is necessary
> to take more into consideration the forces that are present in the
> upper human being tending to a widening, and to the forces present
> in the lower human being, tending to the linear [In this context, the
> gestures of embryonic growth in the cranium and the limbs were
> being considered.] (p. 39).

In every function, both poles are working together. In all rhythmical functions which can be observed directly, the dual nature of lower and upper human being is immediately apparent: in the heartbeat, the upper dominates in the systole, while in the diastole it is the lower human being. The function appears as the result between phases of energy-consuming exertion and up-building recovery. Inhalation is enabled through the upper functions, exhalation through the lower. The mutual, consecutive working of both poles can be seen in all living, rhythmic processes. The rhythmical function may be directly experienced above all in the middle human being. Depolarization is the most important breaking down process in the nerve-sense system. During the depolarization the outer membranes of the nerve cells are opened and salts from the extracellular spaces are absorbed. Repolarization has to immediately restore the integrity of the cell. This double process creates the electrical impulses along the nerves. In the activity of metabolism, the upper human being is revealed in its breaking down of nutritional substance, in excretion and secretion and in energy consumption for movement. The lower human being, on the other hand, builds up again the organism's own substances, its glandular products and its energy-rich substances. However, both processes always appear together rhythmically in reciprocal activity. One side may dominate for a while; the organism, however, will call up the counter-process as quickly as possible. The capacity for rhythmical balancing of polar tendencies is called endogenous regulation. If this is strongly pronounced, the reaction to a strongly breaking down, depleting stimulus can be complete recovery. In the case of an extreme dominance by one or the other process, the organism's short-term capacity for adaptation is insufficient. This leads to temporary overloads of the system, which manifest as illness. In healing, the organism strives to reach a previously unattained, higher degree of adaptation. If one of the two forces becomes permanently one-sided, this ultimately leads to death.

From a threefold point of view, Steiner describes the correlation between the organization of the body and the three soul-processes of thinking, feeling and will. The region of the ether body's living processes is to be found qualitatively between the formed body and the expressions of the soul. All living processes follow a process with a beginning and an end; they are directed toward a goal. They consist in activating and inhibiting impulses, which manifest as rhythmically coordinated. In the course of their activity they call forth their own counter-processes and oscillate rhythmically between an anabolic and a catabolic phase. In the second medical course held parallel to the Eurythmy Therapy Course, the polar arrangement of the upper and lower human being was described in all the lectures. The changing names which Steiner chose depended on the functions being examined. The two forces were called the 'differentiating and synthesizing forces,'[5] the 'arsenizing and albumenizing forces,'[6] the 'building up and breaking down forces,' the 'shaping and dissolving forces,' to mention just some. The same theme is found in the Eurythmy Therapy Course. In the first lecture, the polarity of 'back (upper)' (brain, ear) and 'front (lower)' (larynx, thyroid) appears. The series of these organs, always described in polarity, is completed in the medical course: the upper, back human being consists in the system of processes of brain, lung and liver; the lower, front human being in uterus, heart and larynx. At the same time, the emphasis is less on the anatomy and much more on the processes of these organs. These building up and breaking down processes together form a 'dovetailing of a forward-orientated and a backward-orientated system, [which can] become disjointed (p. 8).

In the sixth lecture of the Eurythmy Therapy Course, it is said that organs could be organically 'too selfless' or 'too wilful'; that they would then have the tendency, on the one hand, to 'dissolve,' or too strongly to form a 'wedge-shape.' Just as in the first lecture of the medical course, the words 'selfless' or 'wilful' do not describe a property of the soul, but point to the quality of a living process: processes which tend toward hardening or which separate themselves distinctly from their surroundings. Attention is drawn to how the upper forces, when they come into contact with existing tissue, on the one hand create structure, on the other bring about hardening or even calcification. The lower forces build up new structures. However, when they act intensively upon existing tissue or organs, their effect is also to dissolve, to deliquesce.

These upper or lower forces can be directly influenced by vocalic and consonantal eurythmy therapy. The rhythmic living forces may be realigned. The whole Eurythmy Therapy Course is composed according to the principle of mutually determining polarities.

In Steiner's work, the polarity of the upper and lower human being is also abbreviated to head or nerve-sense processes on the one hand and metabolic forces on the other. Between these poles he then arranges the respiratory organization and the circulation as mediating systems. In the lecture, 'The Invisible Human Being Within Us,' we also find the collaboration of the direct and indirect processes in the ether body organized from a fourfold aspect. In this fourfolding are reflected the four parts of the human being. This fourfold arrangement of processes is also chosen as the basis for consideration in the Stuttgart Eurythmy Therapy lecture. The hope is there expressed:

These two dynamics [of the upper human being which shapes
and differentiates and of the lower human being which radiates
and correlates with the forces of substances], must be regulated
reciprocally, and one can hope that eurythmy therapists will
cultivate a fine feeling [for this] (p. 116).

The 'eurythmy therapists' are supposed to develop a 'fine feeling' out of the knowledge of the polar organization of processes, in order to become effective therapeutically.

The polarity of the active forces can be extended in a sevenfold differentiation, in order to distinguish the steps of metamorphosis between the poles as life processes, life stages, life movements and so on.[7]

Hans Müller-Wiedemann also draws attention to the importance of the centres of polar forces in the ether body:

Also connected with this is the fundamental knowledge that the
sheaths in the upper and the lower human being work together
in a different manner; thereby a polarity is constituted, the
knowledge of which is just as important for the physician as for
the curative educator and the eurythmy therapist. In the curative
education course this polarity is the subject of Rudolf Steiner's
considerations.[8]

The polar arrangement of the ether body, of the upper and lower human being, is the subject of consideration not only in the curative education course, but in all the medical courses and also the Eurythmy Therapy Course. Ricardo Torriani, too, bases his work on the constitution of the human being on this polarity.

In the present work, the attempt is made to describe the polar arrangement of living processes in such a way that a physiology of eurythmy begins to become perceptible and access to intelligible indications becomes available. Steiner refers frequently to the connection of human formative tendencies with eurythmy therapy: 'You will see now how there is an inward connection between the eurythmical element involved and the human formative tendencies' (p. 42). Elsewhere we find:

This eurythmy therapy works in such a way that the process
arising in normal human life in walking, running and so on –
whereby there are always inner processes involved which are
connected with the human organism's processes of breaking down

and building up – that this process ... works back onto the inner
organs. There are strict rules for this. I can have a person carry
out a system of eurythmy therapy gestures which works back
onto the organism in such a way that, for instance, breaking down
processes which do not want to take their course have now to do
so in the right way; or that, through a different system of eurythmy
therapy, breaking down processes which are acting too strongly are
counteracted accordingly.[9]

Eurythmy therapy should follow 'strict rules.' It should work into
the building up and breaking down forces of the vital body. The aim of
eurythmy therapy is stated:

This is something which brings a great deal of life into this human
etheric body; and in precisely those directions we have pointed
out [eurythmy therapy treatment with vowel and consonant
exercises] ... In these matters, in these exercises the intention
is to bring movement into the human etheric body, to bring an
inwardly regulated movement [between building up and breaking
down processes] into the etheric activity of the human organism.
(pp. 55f).

3. The Polar Effects of Consonants and Vowels

3.1 Characterization of the polar effects in the Eurythmy Therapy Course

The first indication of a differentiated effect of vowels and consonants in eurythmy therapy emerges as early as the second lecture: through doing vowel eurythmy one can treat chronic headaches and migraine. (No particular vowel is named at that point; the Migraine–B exercise is not described until later.) Children, also, who are too bleary can be woken up in this way. The vowel exercises, then, serve to strengthen the impulse to wakefulness; they press back the burgeoning metabolism which manifests in migraine.

The next reference to vowels as cosmic forces which affect embryological formation differently is given in the third lecture: the vowel O works as a form impulse on the necessary broadening of the head, which depends on the regulation of the brain's growth. The vowel E enables the crossing of the nerve pathways. Both these formative impulses are intimately connected with the development of the nervous system. The form impulses which are induced through the other vowels are not mentioned.

In the fourth lecture indications for the consonants are described. They all work on the metabolism and boost the building up forces.

The first systematic differentiation of the effects of consonant and vowel exercises comes in the sixth lecture: making consonants eurythmically counteracts the tendency to become wilful in the soul and organically in the living processes. This 'becoming wilful' manifests in a predominance of the hardening forces, which leads in the long run to crystallization. At the same time a loss of the 'sculptural force' of the 'lower human being' would be apparent. This one-sidedness would lead to a pathological consolidation, to the organs' taking on 'wedge shapes.' Consonantal eurythmy therapy counteracts this tendency to illness through a strengthening of the lower forces. Pulmonary tuberculosis is mentioned in the medical course[1] as an example of this one-sidedness. Later on, Graves' disease is described with the same configuration (in a different place in the organism): once more an organ is shaped too much by the upper forces.[2] The 'wilfulness' manifests clearly in the autonomy of the thyroid nodules. This is the first mention in the Medical course of consonantal eurythmy therapy.

The polar tendency appears when people are organically selfless in a pathological way, when their organs deliquesce. Later on it is said, 'that one is able through vocalic eurythmy ... [to bring] the human being organically to themselves.' Vocalic eurythmy therapy works healingly where the lower human being predominates, because it strengthens the upper forces. This is particularly important for people who remain half asleep through the day; in their case condensing, moulding and consolidating forces need to be strengthened through vocalic exercises. In the Medical Course, a corresponding example of diarrhea is described.[3] Medicinally this should be treated with arsenic. This poison directly strengthens the forces of the upper human being.

In the Eurythmy Therapy Course the imaginative expression 'wedge-form' points to the dominance of the upper human being; at the other pole the danger arises of 'a flowing-out of the organs' through the preponderance of the lower human being.

This rule is maintained until the last lecture of the 1921 course; it gains a higher degree of reality through the exercises in which vowels and consonants are united in a new therapeutic 'word.' In therapy, the sounding together of vocalic and consonantal eurythmy therapy is almost always needed because, even in the most extreme of illnesses, the upper or the lower human being are never working in complete isolation. The therapeutic 'word' practised in eurythmy therapy intervenes in the upper and lower human being and works healingly by way of endogenous regulation.

The soul attribute corresponding to the physiological onesidedness of the upper human being is thinking. On the other hand, the will with its 'chaos of tissue fluidity' correlates with the lower human being.

3.2 Summary

Consonantal eurythmy therapy has a healing effect where there is a dominance of the upper human being:
— when people are too wide awake, where this brings about sleep disturbances
— when organs become too strongly formed by the forces of the head and become 'wedge-shaped'
— when their processes become 'autonomous' and declare their independence from the rest of the organism
— when the functions in individual organs become too strongly hardened and sclerose
— when the body's own substance cannot be built up sufficiently

Vocalic eurythmy therapy has a healing effect where there is a dominance of the lower human being:
— when during the daytime people are too dreamy and consequently become clumsy
— when organs or processes are not able sufficiently to form boundaries between each other
— when processes arise whose time structures are unregulated
— when functions within individual organs work pathologically to dissolve an organ through chronic inflammation processes
— when nutrients cannot completely be transformed and remain a foreign element

In the Eurythmy Therapy Course, therefore, the effect of consonantal eurythmy therapy correlates with a strengthening of the lower human being; that of vocalic eurythmy therapy with a strengthening of the upper human being.

The first description after the Eurythmy Therapy Course confines itself to the speaking of vowels and consonants, 'the vowels give us [in speech] substance, material. The consonants shape what the vowels give as substance.'[4] If speech and eurythmy are understood as polar processes, this indication can be understood with the meaning given until now. For, in the second eurythmy therapy lecture, it is recommended that disturbances of the consonantal element in speech be approached therapeutically with eurythmy therapy vowel exercises.

3.3   Further characterization giving the opposite point of view

In later statements, the eurythmy therapeutic effect of vowels and consonants is initially presented the other way round. In the Stuttgart eurythmy therapy lecture which was held a year and a half after the course, the polarity of the ether body is presented in detail. The forces of the upper human being are here called 'shaping' [*plastizierend*] and 'centripetally' radiating forces (by contrast, the phrase 'plastic [*plastische*] forces' refers mostly to the lower forces which promote growth). Their predominance manifests for example in inhalation; the forces of the lower human being act in a polar opposite direction and predominate in exhalation. The latter are also linked to the processes of substances. The 'forces of exhalation,' which work from below, are strengthened through vocalic eurythmy therapy; the 'shaping forces of inhalation,' by contrast, through consonantal eurythmy therapy. This assertion contrasts with that made in the Eurythmy Therapy Course itself.

The new polar scheme also appears in a notebook entry.[5]

> *Eurythmy*
> *Perception = Consonantal*
> *Will = vocalic*

Perception works in the same way as consonantal eurythmy, which corresponds to the upper human being. The will now correlates with a vocalic effect and is assigned to the lower human being.

This new arrangement is emphasized in further lectures; movements which express vowels strengthen the albumenizing forces. 'Whereas in many cases the antimonizing forces are supported through forces expressing the consonants.'[6] The working of the lower (albumenizing) and the higher (antimonizing) forces is characterized here in the same way as in the notebook entry, but contrary to the description in the Eurythmy Therapy Course.

The same direction of effect is also found in the therapeutic recommendation, 'if it is a question of sclerosis, one would primarily apply vocalic eurythmy therapy ... in the case of inflammatory processes, one would have to employ groups of consonants, namely *L, M, S* and other such sounds.'[7] A predominance of hardening needs to be dissolved vocalically. In all cases of inflammation the lower preponderates and should be therapized through the consonants working from above.

In the Curative Education Course as well consonants are used in order to strengthen the arsenizing forces. This arsenizing is identical to the catabolic intervention of the day/astral body. The child should do consonantal eurythmy therapy (*R, L, M, N*); the effect can be intensified through arsenic.[8] For a child with kleptomania, vocalic eurythmy therapy with the legs is later recommended, because this 'drives the intellectual element out of the will and the endeavour lying in the vowels into the will.'[9] By the same token a child with memory loss, in whom 'the upper organism' is not effective enough 'in the lower organism,' is therapized through *L, M, S* and *U*.[10] Once more, consonantal eurythmy therapy strengthens the breaking down forces of the upper human being. However, a boy in whom the 'inhalation process outweighs the exhalation process' (in whom therefore the upper human being is working too strongly) was brought to better exhalation (lower human being) through *M*.[11]

In other, later lectures, the efficacy of consonants and vowels is once more presented in terms of the original description; in the course for young physicians it is explained that consonantal eurythmy therapy corresponds to the forces of the moon.[12] These allow the long bones to grow up 'out of the earth' from within and below. Shaping, building up forces and hidden, building up sculptors are at work here. In a polar opposite way, vocalic eurythmy therapy corresponds to the Saturn forces. These shape the cranium from above and without. One can observe concretely these forces of Saturn, which work from the outer world, when finger nails are cut. (This indication on the working of moon-forces is the opposite of the one in the Eurythmy Therapy Course. In the third lecture (p. 39) the moon activity is described in terms of the moon's effecting the 'widening' of the head.)

In a different medical lecture the original correlation appears once more: vocalic eurythmy therapy was to be done in the case of a patient with sleep disorders and compulsive thought processes.[13] It was said that with these symptoms the will was trapped too much in the head and needed to be guided back into the limbs. In other words the lower, will human being was to be guided back into a healthy balance by strengthening the upper forces (through vocalic eurythmy therapy).

In the last reference to the polar effects of vowel and consonant, vocalic eurythmy therapy was recommended when salts or carbohydrates from food too strongly maintained their foreign, external form tendency. The 'upper forces' were not strong enough to overcome the foreignness. The result was that the nutritional substances could not sufficiently be internalized.[14] At this point, the presentation is once more in accordance with the Eurythmy Therapy Course: vocalic eurythmy therapy strengthens the forces of the 'upper human being.'

In the book, *Fundamentals of Therapy*, a whole chapter is devoted to eurythmy therapy, although the effect is not differentiated as to vowels and consonants.

3.4   Description of the polar effects in subsequent literature

In the literature on eurythmy therapy, the issue of the different descriptions of the effects of vocalic and consonantal eurythmy therapy appears most clearly in the work of Ursula Steinke. The author wrestles with these contrasting descriptions in her *Lesebuch Heileurythmie*, writing, 'If one goes deeper into such an enumeration [of the effects of vocalic and consonantal eurythmy therapy], one is struck immediately by the apparent contradictions.' She focuses in some detail on albumenizing as a function of the lower human being, and goes on to describe 'condensing or strengthening the self' (which is a function of the upper human being) as an effect of the vowels. She does not come to a satisfactory resolution of the contradiction.

Klaus Höller describes the effect of vowels and consonants as they appear in the Eurythmy Therapy Course but without clearly stating the issue of divergent descriptions. Eduardo Jenaro gives a similar characterization: '[The vowels] induce a consolidation of the aura and act with an incarnating gesture on the human being, strengthening the self.' In early books, like Margarete Kirchner-Bockholt's *Foundations of Curative Eurythmy*, and Julia Bort's *Heileurythmie mit seelenpflege-bedürftigen Kindern*, the question is not addressed.

3.5   Attempts to resolve the contradiction

To sum up, the following can be said: in the lectures in the Eurythmy Therapy Course, vocalic eurythmy therapy is shown to strengthen the 'wedge-shape forming' upper forces; and consonantal eurythmy therapy to strengthen the building up activity and the dissolving tendency within it. In the medical lectures up to January 1924 and in the curative education course the portrayal is reversed; vocalic eurythmy therapy now strengthens the lower, albumenizing forces. Only in the last lectures is the original correlation re-established: vocalic eurythmy therapy strengthens the human being's upper forces, which are necessary for breaking down foreign nutritional forces. Consonantal eurythmy therapy strengthens the lower forces which bring about building up.

The problem we have described, of the differing indications for the direction of efficacy accorded to vocalic and consonantal eurythmy therapy, is further confused in that Steiner over and again describes the 'rhythmical system' as the place where vowels are effective. 'The vowels in eurythmy work ... directly on the rhythmic organism. With the consonantal eurythmical movements the case is that, although the rhythmic organism is, of course, also affected, this is accomplished by way of the system of the metabolism and limbs.' (p. 46). Two days earlier Steiner had presented to the physicians in detail that in the middle, rhythmical human being only the 'effects of the lower human being and the effects of the upper human being are at play.'[15] Therefore the statement made in this quotation must logically be supplemented as follows: 'the vowels in eurythmic activity work ... [from the nerve-sense system, the upper human being] directly onto the rhythmical organism.'

No adequate solution to the contradictory accounts has yet been found. One possible explanation could arise if Steiner had wanted different phases of therapy to be dealt with differently. The necessity for opposite strategies over the course of an illness can be described by taking therapy for a fever as an example: when the fever is rising, the patient freezes in bouts of shivering. They need help from extra blankets and hot-water bottles in order to warm up. After the fever reaches its peak opposite therapeutic measures are called for: the warm covers are removed and cooling poultices applied. It is particularly emphasized in the medical course that with every therapy one has to reckon with a direct effect from the therapeutic agent and with a polar reaction from the organism. Whether the principle of polar therapeutic approach is sufficient to resolve the contradiction mentioned above must remain open.

A different point of view for resolving the contradiction would arise if eurythmy therapy with children and with adults had to be carried out in opposite ways. With children the soul and the I are still working from the periphery and not yet incarnated in the body. The next step in the incarnation of the I is characterized in the parallel medical course in the following way. The unconscious I lives in the periphery of the body roughly until the ninth year. From this time 'this I [is] given birth in an inward direction as well [into the metabolism].'[16] This 'inward birth' is an essential precondition for the I's being able to take a last step into the exoteric: the age of responsibility is reached. These three phases of activity of the same I organization, differing from each other in principle, could also explain the differing indications for the way eurythmy therapy works. Admittedly there is no textual basis for these thoughts. On the contrary, there are many places where children and adults are mentioned with the same illness and the same therapy (for instance in connection with the I-exercise in the second lecture).

No satisfactory solution has yet been found by any of the eurythmy therapists and physicians whom we have asked. In order, however, to reach a working proposition – which may be corrected later – the arrangement which first appeared in the Eurythmy Therapy Course will continue to be used. This decision is supported by the repetition of this arrangement in the last lectures.

In summary, we therefore conclude that consonantal eurythmy therapy strengthens the lower, building up processes in the human being, while vocalic eurythmy therapy supports the activity of the upper, breaking down and forming forces in the whole organism.

4. The Three Elements of Eurythmy

4.1 Rudolf Steiner's first description of movement, feeling and character

Eurythmy had its first beginnings in 1911: the mother of Lory Maier-Smits enquired about a profession for her daughter in the world of movement. Lory Maier-Smits became the first eurythmist, and over the next few years eurythmy developed out of anthroposophy as a new art of movement, making its appearance in performances as speech eurythmy and music eurythmy. Both aspects were at first built up purely out of artistic activity. Only eleven years later were the artistic elements presented conceptually in comparison to the other arts in a lecture.[1] The basic elements of sculpture were described as the taut, shaped surfaces of forms in space, those of painting as colour, luminance and form on the surface of the base material. Thus each art had its own medium in which to shape and realize itself. The basic elements of eurythmy were then described:

> The human being's limb movements, particularly those of the arms
> and hands but also what appears everywhere in the movement
> of the whole human body, are the primary means of expression
> of the art of eurythmy. 'Movement' itself is therefore what we
> need to consider in the first place. ... This movement can only
> appear as ensouled, if the eurythmists also have the 'feeling' that
> they themselves feel this 'movement' with their own movement;
> as if there were some tangible air up here which felt different to
> normal air ... Imagine them moving their arm like this and feeling
> something either touching and pushing them gently or maybe
> pulling them ... Then the spectator can see what the eurythmist
> feels, inasmuch as the latter can really shape and place the veil
> so skilfully that one can see that they feel a slight pressure here
> or a gentle tug there ... [This feeling of the slight pressure or the
> gentle tug, is to be] poured into the shape of the veil while moving
> eurythmically.

Alongside the movement and the feeling of eurythmy, the element embodying the will, the 'character' of the gesture, is then described. The character is experienced as a tensing of the muscles, as something that is felt as the development of a force in the muscles. This tensing arises in different places within the body, according to the different sounds:

> You tauten your forehead for a particular letter or passage that you are presenting; or with a particular movement you feel you are strengthening the muscles of the upper arm; or you consciously position your feet while pressing down onto the floor when doing another movement. This is the third element, 'character.'

It is emphasized that everything can be expressed through the three elements of movement, feeling and character:

> Everything which eurythmy intends to achieve artistically ... is nothing more than movement, feeling and character as I have described them. Just as the sculptor controls the surfaces, the reciter shapes the sounds and the musician the tones, in order to achieve their purpose, so too the eurythmist must achieve everything that can be attained, using movement, feeling and character. Nothing further may be considered. This is the realm of eurythmy's artistic media. With these media everything must be accomplished.

What stands out in this quotation is its exclusive nature: no other possible elements are acceptable in accomplishing the art of eurythmy; everything depends on taking hold of eurythmy with these media.

These three elements are mentioned repeatedly in later lectures. But only in this lecture are the artistic elements of eurythmy characterized as pure sense perceptions. These crucial statements therefore need to be emphasized again.

1. Movement

> The first thing that needs to be considered is movement itself. The spectator can only experience eurythmy in its entirety when they can behold something in movement as such: in the movement which is accorded to a vowel or a consonant, for example, or in the formation of a gesture which arises from the movement. ... Let us imagine that the movement for a particular letter makes the eurythmist move their arm like this and then halt briefly. This is the movement. [This movement is drawn on the blackboard.]

2. Feeling

> This movement will only give the effect of being imbued with soul if the eurythmist additionally has the feeling that they perceive this movement with their own gesture in such a way that here above them there is some tangible air which feels different to the rest of

the air ... They move their arm like this and feel something very gently touching and pressing them or something else tugging them ... The spectator then sees ... how the eurythmist feels the gentle pressure here or light tug there.

In another lecture we find the following:

When you see the eurythmist on stage controlling their veil, it is essentially a continuation of the movement. This development continues in such a way that at the appropriate moment there is a wafting or a billowing of the veil; a thorough configuration of the veil. Thus the movement carried out through the limbs lives in what is expressed as feeling in the handling of the veil ... If the eurythmist feels the right element in the gesture made by their arms and legs, it will instinctively be carried over into their handling of the veil; then, in the way they handle the veil, they will have the feeling that ought to accompany the gesture.[2]

3. Character

You tauten your forehead for a particular letter or passage that you are presenting; or with a particular gesture you feel you are bringing energy into the muscles of the upper arm; or you consciously position your feet while pressing down on the floor when doing another movement. That is the third element, 'character.'

In a later lecture the elements were demonstrated using the figures:

So that the muscle here in the forehead is particularly tautened and here in the neck as well, while here the muscles remain freer and more relaxed. The eurythmist can distinguish very accurately whether they are moving their arm outward in a relaxed way, or whether they are tensing the muscle inwardly. Through this muscular tension which is felt by the eurythmist, character is brought into the eurythmy ... The moment the eurythmist reveals a charming facial expression, it no longer has anything to do with creating eurythmy; the latter can come about only through what the eurythmist is able to make of their face by bringing muscular tension into it.[3]

In one of the teachers'meetings at the Waldorf School, Steiner said following about 'character': 'For example, when doing eurythmic movements, the eurythmist must feel the pressure from one limb onto the other and the counterflow of the pressure back into the centre of the body.'[4]

4.1.1 Perception of movement, feeling and character

The three elements of movement underlie eurythmy. In the lectures, the word 'movement' has two meanings. Sometimes it describes the totality of movement; on other occasions the individual element movement. The individual element is the easiest to grasp: it describes the flow of a movement as it appears. This individual element is seen at its clearest in the uniformly flowing movement of an arm. In the process as little effort as possible should be put into the flow of the movement. Another aspect of the movement element has to do with the spatial direction into which the eurythmic gesture is formed; it can swing out into all three spatial dimensions.

Movement is perceived predominantly through the sense of movement. Every movement creates a greater or lesser imbalance of the body which our sense of movement immediately detects. This prompts the organism unconsciously to modify the muscle tone in the corresponding parts of the body, so that balance is maintained. The pure movement element leads to fatigue only after a long while. This is then perceived by the sense of life.

Character is described as the counter-pole to movement: the muscles should tighten and develop energy. This unfolding of energy should be felt in the body. In the natural course of movement, muscular force is felt in every rapid acceleration or deceleration of a movement and in every stance which is held for long. It is even possible to observe the different degrees of basic tension underlying the muscles during a uniform movement: it can be executed with too much or too little tension.

Character is also perceived with the help of the sense of movement. In addition fatigue sets in as a result of the muscular tension more quickly than in the case of movement; the sense of life comes into action. The fatigue can be felt in individual groups of muscles or in the whole body. If the strong activity of the muscles is maintained for long, a general warming can be experienced.

Feeling, as well, is described as a primary perception of the senses: the pressure and suction of the surrounding air should be felt; the experience of being touched delicately by something from the periphery becomes conscious. This perception should inform the guiding of the veil.

> If the eurythmist can feel the right thing in the movement into
> which they bring their arms and legs, then this movement they
> feel will quite instinctively pass into the handling of the veil; and
> they will have in the treatment of the veil the feeling that should
> accompany the movement.[5]

The main thing is the perception of the pressure or suction of the surrounding air. This is perceived through the sense of touch. Through this perception the eurythmist is able to direct the veil appropriately, awakening the right experience in the spectator.

An experience of pressure or suction can be experienced in a much more elementary way if movements are made in water or during a storm. If the arm is spread out, the airflow from the back is dammed up against the back of the hand and the outside of the forearm. At the same time a gentle suction may be felt on the other side. This sensory experience in the body can be termed feeling. At the same time, the eurythmist experiences in their soul that, in the course of the same spreading movement, their arms are sucked out into the periphery, where the damming of the air can be experienced as a pure sensory perception. It is a polar experience: on the one hand the sense perception (the damming of the air outside while spreading the arm); on the other, the soul experience that the arm is sucked out into the periphery. The veil reveals this duality: as the movement of the arms spreads out, it flutters in the opposite direction and draws together.

The perception of feeling again occurs through the will-senses: the senses of movement, of balance and of life; the senses of touch and of warmth are also involved. After all, pressure and suction are experienced through touch; the localization of pressure is experienced through a certain cooling, that of suction as a warming, if the air is cooler than one's own hand.

At this point, the dual meaning of the word feeling needs to be addressed. People 'feel' with their sense of touch whether a surface is rough or smooth. They 'feel' with their sense of life whether they are tired. They feel whether they have lost their balance through a sudden movement; they 'feel' the flow of their arm's movement with their sense of movement or position. Our language uses the word 'feel' for the perceptions that are made through all four lower senses (senses of the will) and through the sense of warmth. The word points to the sensory experience of one's own body in relation to the environment.

It is important to differentiate clearly from these the 'feeling' within the soul in which sympathy and antipathy are experienced in relation to sensory experience. In the initial description of the elements movement, feeling and character, 'sensing feeling' is referred to throughout, not 'soul feeling.' For the primary perception of eurythmy, the eurythmist has to direct their attention to all the lower senses: in movement and character the senses of movement, balance and life predominate; for feeling they are joined by those of touch and warmth. Perception in relation to one's own body forms the basis of eurythmy.

4.1.2   Synaesthetic perceptions of movement, feeling and character

During subsequent presentations of the coloured wooden eurythmy figures, the experiencing of the three elements in one's own body through
the will-senses is expanded in three ways.

First, the three elements are represented in the figures in particular
forms: movement appears as the whole form or 'dress'; feeling is shown
spatially on the figure as the 'veil'; character is accentuated in particular
areas, its identity appearing through the accentuated areas. When one
observes the eurythmy figures, the form of the three elements is perceived
primarily by the sense of the word or gestalt. With eurythmic movements
themselves, however, it is likely that differentiated formal perception of
the three individual elements is possible only in a primary way for the
trained observer.

Secondly, the three elements are made visible in the figures through
colour. The comment is made:

> Eurythmy avails itself of those artistic media with which one can
> actually create artistically forms of expression in the 'movement'
> of the human body and in the 'feeling' and 'character' that are
> poured into the limbs. ... Following these principles, sounds
> ... are handled in such a way that one gives each sound its due
> through a certain manner of expression, so that the movement is
> really brought out in one colouring, the feeling in another and the
> character comes to expression in a third colour ...'[6]

In the figures, the three colours are always given as a direct (primary)
perception. In eurythmic movement, however, this sense-bound colour
perception vanishes. It emerges by contrast as a synaesthetic perception
in the eurythmist and in the observer. This is described below in more
detail.

Thirdly, the third extension of the primary sense experience arises
when the three elements are correlated with the three soul gestures of
thinking, feeling and will. The movement element, which always appears
spatially and which can be most consciously experienced, is grasped with
thinking; the feeling of pressure or suction, of warmth or cold, points to
the soul content of feeling; and the tensing of the musculature in character
lets the will become conscious.

The representation of the sounds in the figures through form and
colour has the aim 'on one hand that one can be brought to an understanding of eurythmy and on the other that the eurythmists themselves
will also be able to learn a great deal from these representations, in that
having the figurative representation in front of them gives them the

essential aspects of any eurythmic element.'[7] The eurythmist should learn the essence of a eurythmic sound, which is built up primarily from the three individual elements movement, feeling and character, through the forms and colours of the figures by practising and through thinking. The figures are merely an aid to bring what we see of the movement to a higher experience. The path to this 'making the invisible visible' consists in consciously extending the senses on which eurythmic activity is based.

Sense experiences are mediated through the senses: the temperature of an object is perceived through the sense of warmth; colours, brightness and darkness through the sense of sight. Both are just as much primary or direct sense experiences of the environment as the 'feeling' of eurythmy through the sense of movement or of an imbalance through the sense of balance. Primary sense experiences mediate the experience of the physical sense-world.

In all artistic activities, there are experiences which go beyond this which are no longer susceptible of sense perception, but which possess a high degree of general validity: a high note can sound 'bright' and 'sharp'; a colour is experienced as 'warm' or 'cold'; a movement as 'red in colour.' This activity of secondary sense experience Steiner calls sensory symbiosis.[8] In general literature this phenomenon is usually described as synaesthetic experience.

Sensory symbioses appear within all perceptions. The experience, however, only becomes conscious and more certain through schooling. The more one practises and differentiates consciously these secondary experiences, the more vivid the primary perceptions become. The resonating experiences are no longer pure sensory ones. They point, in fact, to a supersensible experience which is related to an imagination. The spectra of primary sense experiences and the significance of the symbiotic (synaesthetic) experiences for all the arts, but particularly for eurythmy, were elaborated by Thomas Göbel:

> In all the arts mentioned we have been able to discover sensory
> symbioses as part of the enjoyment of art. But they are consciously
> cultivated only in eurythmy. Without such a practice, artists are
> living in the world of sensory symbioses as if in a dream. Waking
> up to it is a step demanded of us by the spirit of our time.[9]

At this point it is important to highlight a clear distinction between primary and secondary experiences during eurythmic activity. The basis of eurythmy is the primary perception of the three individual elements movement, feeling and character. To experience this foundation consciously calls for a training of the will-senses during eurythmic practice. In a first intensification, the primary experience is extended to an experience of sensory symbioses. In the experience of the colour of movement, feeling and character, imagination awakens half-consciously. This stage in the extension of consciousness is called by Steiner the 'enlivening of the sensory processes.'

A further, still higher transformation of experience is described in the same lecture as 'ensouling of the life-processes.' Here consciousness is directed to the question as to which impulses arise in the thinking, feeling and acting soul when a primary sense experience is made. 'What the life-organs otherwise unfold by way of sympathetic and antipathetic forces is as it were instilled again into the sense organs. The eye not only sees the red, it also feels sympathy or antipathy for the colour.'[10] The 'ensouling of the life processes' points to the process whereby impulses of thought, sympathetic or antipathetic feelings, and impulses of the will resonate, largely unconsciously, in all sensory experience. The primary sensory experience of the movement element is extended in this spirit, in the description of the eurythmy figures, to the effect that attention to movement most clearly mediates impulses of thought. When taking in character, which is experienced through muscular tension, the human being's will resonates.

Primary experience of the environment, which during movement is based on the perception of pressure and suction on the surface of and around the arm, is called feeling. We have already drawn attention to the difference between 'perceptual feeling' (I feel the roughness of a surface) and 'soul feeling' (I feel my delight as I touch the surface). There is a third quality of 'feeling.' For example, if one has cogitated for a long time on a problem, a feeling begins to appear in the soul after a while that can be described broadly as follows, 'I feel that my search has brought me close to a solution. I don't have the solution yet, but I do have a definite feeling that it will soon be possible to formulate it.' Similarly a feeling can live in us as to whether a decision or a resolve is the right one. This quality of feeling is very delicate and always directed to a future in which something needs to come about.

With the word feeling, therefore, three realms must always be distinguished: 'perceptual feeling' kindles in the touching of a finished object; inner 'soul-feeling' arises with every human experience, always spontaneously and immediately, as sympathy or antipathy; the 'feeling for something coming into being' concentrates an inkling within, which points to future cognition or knowledge. Whether the intuited solution to a scientific problem is really sustainable can only ever be judged later. The 'feeling for something coming into being,' when it is consciously sought after, conveys a high degree of inner evidence. It opens the soul for unresolved challenges which need to be taken up through thinking and acting.

Sensory perception of what surrounds one, experienced consciously in 'feeling,' opens the eurythmist's soul for this 'feeling for something coming into being.'

Every primary sense-experience can be tested in this way for impulses to think, feel and act which lie below the surface and which resonate during perception. The more strongly these become conscious, the clearer it becomes that the accompanying experiences that arise go beyond the level of imagination. They are echoes of inspiration, which resonate in the doing and experiencing of eurythmy.

The three basic elements, movement, feeling and character, should express everything in eurythmy. The first, most comprehensive presentation by Rudolf Steiner describes the primary perceptions which should be practiced through the will-senses during eurythmy. On this foundation the colour and soul experiences which are the symbioses of the senses then gain their higher reality.

4.1.3   Summary

Eurythmy's three elements – movement, feeling and character – are described by Steiner initially as primary sense experiences. The eurythmist should become conscious of their own movements through the four senses of the will, in order to practise each individual movement element in the spirit of an étude and thereby to increase their eurythmic ability. Movement, the flow of movement; character, the experience of energy; and feeling, the experience of the periphery, are sensorily perceptible. Through a trained 'enlivening' of these sense experiences, the movements of the sounds can be experienced imaginatively anew in their threefold colour. The next step, of 'ensouling,' establishes the connection of the three elements with the impulses of thinking, feeling and acting. Precursors of inspiration can become conscious for the eurythmist. The elements of the eurythmy of the sounds thus become elements of practice which lead from the sensory world into supersensible reality.

4.2   Movement, feeling and character in the Eurythmy Therapy Course

The Eurythmy Therapy Course was given a good year before the first presentation of eurythmy's three basic elements, so this differentiation was not yet referred to. Descriptions of the elements are clearly discernible in some places; in others they may be sensed. Some examples follow.

1. Reference is made in many places to the effect that the muscles can be felt during eurythmy therapy exercises. This can be read as a clear allusion to character.
2. 'What is essential in artistic eurythmy ... is not the mere form of the limb in position seen from without [that is, the movement], but that which comes into being when the stretching or the bending within the positioned limb is *felt*. What is felt in the limb is what is important.' (p. 11).
3. The most difficult to find in the Eurythmy Therapy Course as a separate element is feeling. Perhaps the following statement is relevant in this respect. 'These three principles of classification: [1] vocalic tingeing, [2] blowing, impacting ... and [3] all that is connected with this external classification [of the teeth, lip and palatal sounds] come to expression in the forms that are there for making eurythmy.' These three 'principles of classification' should be just as visible in eurythmy as are the three elements movement, feeling and character in the later description.

A conscious modification of the three basic elements in moving from eurythmy to eurythmy therapy is decisive for the success of eurythmy therapy and for the health of the eurythmy therapist.

Precisely in this area we have to maintain a strict separation between the goals which we pursue in salutogenesis and therapy and that artistic quality which we have to strive to attain in eurythmy. Anyone who persists in mixing the two will first of all ruin their artistic ability in eurythmy, and secondly find themselves unable to achieve anything of importance in respect to its salutogenic and therapeutic element.' (p. 2).

The quality of a gesture should be described completely and exclusively through the conceptual designation of movement, feeling and character. These elements should have been acquired in eurythmy and taken hold of anew in pedagogical and therapeutic eurythmy.

The change transforming artistic into pedagogical eurythmy, is referred to in teachers' meetings. Evidently clashes had previously taken place. This led to Steiner's commenting on the difference between gymnastics and eurythmy.

It will be appreciated that no clash with eurythmy is intended, if one just considers 'character' in pedagogical eurythmy – which has happened far too little, because it comes less into consideration in artistic performance, whereas in the pedagogical it comes into consideration quite particularly. ... 'Movement' and 'feeling' are going quite well, which up till now is nearly all that has been considered. By contrast, the nature of 'character' in eurythmic

movement has not yet been penetrated. It is quite natural that it has
not yet been penetrated, because it is not of such great importance
in eurythmy's artistic elaboration, where it is viewed by other
people. Hence the 'character' of a movement must form an
essential element in the didactic.[11]

He suggested that much more weight needs to be given to 'character'
in pedagogical eurythmy – but 'it has not yet been penetrated [by euryth-
mists].' Emphasis on the element of 'character' is even more essential in
the progression from eurythmy to eurythmy therapy.

Eurythmy therapy itself was to be gradually modified. In one of the
teachers' meetings, on Steiner's being asked whether even deformities
can be treated through eurythmy therapy, the following answer was given.

Eurythmy therapy was initially elaborated by me as a system
... and this eurythmy therapy is intended in the first place to
contribute to different healing processes. ... It is however the case
that what is needed for lesser deformities [illnesses] lies within
what has already been given as eurythmy therapy. For more severe
deformities it will be a case of intensifying or modifying things in
some way.'[12]

So eurythmy therapy should be intensified or modified in some way
if the process of an illness was more developed or a chronic disability
existed. Such a modification can be introduced only through altering one
or all of the elements movement, feeling and character.

In order consciously to metamorphose the movements from artistic
eurythmy into an effective eurythmy therapy, three questions arise.

1. How can the eurythmy therapist transform and intensify their movement in order that this element in the patient be assessed rightly?
2. How can the eurythmy therapist work with the feeling of the sound-
movements in order to be therapeutically effective.
3. How can the eurythmy therapist perceive character in themselves in
such a way that the patient comes to a sufficient level of experience
without being thrown back too soon on their own muscular tension?

4.3 Other descriptions of movement, feeling and character

Clarification of which areas of experience and what nexus of thought are
included in the three concepts movement, feeling and character is certainly not yet complete. Quotations follow from some authors who have
worked with this question.

The representation of movement, feeling and character as basic
elements of eurythmic movement is described by Eduardo Jenaro. For

movement, he emphasises the 'flowing stream of movement, ... which ... determines the particular relationship ... of the gestures to levity or weight.' Movement is 'the etheric-bodily basis of the movement of the sound.' Feeling is 'its plenitude of soul,' and character gives 'the whole movement of the sound its configuration of time.' Jenaro relates the three basic elements of eurythmy only to a certain extent to primary sensory experiences through the four bodily senses.

In his essay Werner Barfod takes the metamorphosis of speaking and moving as his starting-point. For speech, he pursues the trinity of dynamic, which transforms into the movement of eurythmy; of voicing, which becomes the feeling; and articulation, which corresponds to the character of eurythmy. He does not differentiate between vowel and consonant; he takes as an example the impact sound K. He describes how 'the initiating will impulse always stands at the beginning of a movement, even when a thought provides the stimulus; it is the will which takes hold of [the thought].' For all visible movements, the elements movement, feeling and character always appear in this order, according to his description. From this and other details, it becomes apparent that he has investigated the three elements according to their artistic and supersensible reality, rather than their perceptual content accessible through the senses.

Thomas Parr's description of the three elements remains general:
The nature of the movement in space is expressed through the eurythmy garments. Through the costume, the degree of liveliness with which speech and music are shaped becomes 'movement.' This determines in the first instance the relation of the vertical to the human figure. ... This [movement] becomes imbued with soul as it is experienced as movement. The veil in eurythmy shapes the mood and the feeling for the coming into existence of a gesture.'[13]

He does not elucidate in what manner the element of movement needs to be modified in order to express the element of feeling in the right way. Steiner's repeated indications to the effect that the perception of suction and pressure from the surroundings should be experienced in the element feeling are not taken up in Parr's accounts.

5. Eurythmy and
Other Movement Therapies

In this chapter we shall only touch on physiotherapy (or therapeutic gymnastics) and dance therapy alongside eurythmy therapy. We shall attempt to look at other movement therapies with the same three criteria as eurythmy. For the elements movement, feeling and character can be sought and evaluated in all movement. One's own perception of the flow of movement, experience of muscular tension and observing of peripheral forces can be practiced with all movements. Along with being able to discriminate between these qualities, therapists from the different movement therapies can begin to understandeach other. The perceptions of these three elements are a common foundation. Sensations of form and colour that also resonate in eurythmy, are unfamiliar to physiotherapists and dance therapists. The synaesthetic soul experiences which resonate during movement are verbalized in dance therapy.

5.1 Physiotherapy (therapeutic gymnastics)

In the physiology of movement one distinguishes two kinds of muscular contraction as the basis of all movements of the voluntary muscles: isotonic and isometric contractions. Both types (nearly) always appear together in natural movements; in their systematics, and as far as their therapeutic indications are concerned, they are clearly distinguishable. Through the isotonic contraction of a group of muscles, a movement with a uniform, flowing course and the least possible effort of energy arises. The word 'isotonic' refers to the tendency to keep the muscular tension (tone) as even (iso-) as possible, while attaining the greatest possible contraction. The movement proceeds uniformly and without sudden changes of direction. As an example of such a movement one might move the forearm horizontally to and fro, effortlessly. The lengths of the muscles change, but the muscular tension remains largely the same.

The opposite is isolated isometric contraction. Here the movement is restricted while the muscular tension is increased. For instance, holding a bucket in the same place with one's arm bent and letting it slowly fill with water, shows that the force must continually be increased while there is almost no movement. The metrics (the measurable extent of movement) remains the same (iso); the tone is altered. Human movements are usually a varying combination of both parts. When a new movement is learnt, too much energy is expended and the amount of energy is not yet adapted to the result. In every practised sequence of movements, only as much energy and flow is given to it as is necessary for the outcome of the work. This form of movement, adapted to its purpose, is called auxotonic contraction.

One essential task of physiotherapy is to re-establish the normal mobility of the body, where this has been reduced or has ceased completely. The aim here is to improve the degree of freedom of the joints, the functionality of the joint capsules, ligaments and tendons, and the strength of the musculature through passive or progressively intensified active training. By optimizing movement processes it is possible to promote secondary therapeutic effects in other organ functions.

Treatment for lumbago by means of exercises may be taken as an example. Mobility of the spine, the ability to stand upright and to walk are painfully restricted. Headaches and breathing disorders or other symptoms in different parts of the body can subsequently arise. The main concern is to reduce pain and restore or improve local mobility. Massage therapy may initially be necessary to restore the function of the spine. The aim here is to relax groups of muscles which have gone into spasm. The normal functions of the spine should be restored as soon as possible through active movement therapy. Isometric and isotonic exercises for the limbs and torso are essential therapeutic measures. The therapist first exercises areas of movement which are not directly affected in order then to approach the pathological blockage. Then the groups of muscles that are particularly affected may be approached. Additionally the patient should acquire the ability to practise their programme of exercises daily.

In neuro-physiological exercise therapy (as represented by Bobath, Vojta etc.) the issue broadens: here it is not just a matter of improving the mobility of a joint or the interplay of joints, ligaments and muscles. Through these exercise therapies, the aim is to intensify the integration of synapses and the development of certain regions of the brain toward maturity, so that a return to normal functioning occurs. The exercises have as their starting point a training in movement for the limbs. It is however not only the functions of joints and muscles that are built up but, beyond that, the control of neuro-muscular movement. Ergotherapy (occupational and work therapy) also uses playful exercise-based schooling of movement, with the goal of reconstituting auxotonic processes or establishing new ones in order to compensate.

In the Eurythmy Therapy Course, gymnastics is mentioned three times. Gymnastics is characterized as follows: 'Normal gymnastic movements are in reality taken from the physiology, from the *physis* of the body alone' (p. 66). Important indications for the differentiation of the elements movement, feeling and character in gymnastics and eurythmy are given in one of the teachers' meetings.[1] Physiotherapy can be characterized in exactly the same way. In this movement therapy, processes of healing are to be activated from within the anatomy and physiology of the body. This has the advantage that the gymnastics therapist directs their treatment according to clear diagnoses and can apply their skills appropriately. A danger arises if the patient, through insufficient guidance, carries out the exercises mechanically. Mechanical movements carry the risk of becoming independent and no longer being intended and controlled by the human being. This danger is exacerbated if the client simultaneously reads or is distracted by a film during the exercises. It can then happen that early symptoms of overload go unnoticed and muscles or ligaments can be damaged or torn. There is an indication about this risk: the building up processes of the ether body are no longer able to follow the course of the movement. 'The physical body then does its own movements which do *not* pull after them the movements of the etheric body in the corresponding manner' (p. 66).

For eurythmy therapy the following should be borne in mind:
    What we are developing as artistic eurythmy can unite with
    what is developed as physiological gymnastics. One can make
    the transition from the eurythmical to the gymnastic quite well.
    (pp. 53f).

Eurythmy therapy and appropriate physiotherapy may be done by a patient at the same time. In that case it is helpful to be aware of the common basis of different movement therapies.

It is easy to see that the same movement phenomena are described in therapeutic gymnastics and in eurythmy therapy. The physiology of muscles calls the flowing movement that arises with a minimum of energy isotonic contraction. Steiner differentiates the three elements movement, feeling and character within every movement (Chapter 4). He does not look at the individual muscle but at the flow of a human movement. The element movement corresponds here to the flowing, effortless movement of the body, which manifests in space and time. Isotonic contraction predominates in this element of movement; energy plays only a subordinate role. This aspect is the basis of all facial expression, every gesture and every movement. The eurythmic element movement allows a flowing, effortless movement picture to arise.

Tensing of the muscles is an isometric aspect. The development of force within movement is described and experienced in eurythmy as character. A predominance of character would be expressed in a taut and powerful, minimal flow of movement in which isometric contractions predominate.

In physiotherapy, attention to the isotonic and isometric aspects of movement is crucial; the eurythmic element feeling, that is the experience of the periphery, is not consciously practised. Therapeutic gymnastics and eurythmy therapy have in common that they are based on the isotonic movements and isometric character aspects of the course of an action. An essential difference between both kinds of movement is that in eurythmy the feeling, that is the experience of the periphery, has to be included and shaped. In artistic eurythmy, the experience of feeling is enhanced through the movement of the veil in the surrounding air. In eurythmy therapy, this resource is seldom utilized. It is all the more important that the primary perception of feeling has been schooled in the therapist, so that this element also lives in the therapy.

> For the other kinds of gymnastics take into account ... the
> materialistic prejudices of our time and tend to take their starting
> point from the bodily aspect. The bodily aspect is also taken into
> account in eurythmy. But body, soul and spirit work together in
> eurythmy, so that in eurythmy one has an ensouled and spirit-
> imbued gymnastics.[2]

The elements movement and character characterize the movement therapies which are based on purely muscular activity. Only when attention is directed consciously to the periphery, which is a part of movement, does the dimension of ensoulment and imbuing-with-spirit arise. From the quotation it becomes clear that great importance is attached to the systematic schooling of the primary sensory experiences of the elements movement, feeling and character in the training of the eurythmist. If primary perception via the will-senses is enhanced through sensory symbioses to imaginative colour perceptions and inspirational experiences of the soul's impulses, soul and spirit will live actively in movement. The experience of the pressure and suction of the surrounding air during movement forms thereby the basis for a perception of feeling. From this the sensory symbiotic experience of form and colour elements can develop. Through this the human being trains themself in order to awaken for the ensouling of movement and the imbuing of it with spirit.

5.2   Dance therapy

A completely different approach is adopted by dance therapy. It is a new form of therapy in which movements from other cultural backgrounds are deployed as a means to healing. Gisela Bräuner-Gülow and Helge Gülow first described the connection of eurythmy therapy to dance therapy, writing, 'From the viewpoint of eurythmy therapy, using basic general concepts, interesting parallels [to dance therapy] arise initially. But closer examination shows when and where the differences crop up.' The 'basic general concepts' they have in common are the three elements movement, feeling and character, even if this is not brought out in their writing. We have used *Healing Movement* by Reitz and others for the description of dance therapy.

The therapeutic forms in dance therapy and drama therapy have developed, not from somatic medicine, but from psychotherapy. One paradigm of this therapy is the assumption 'that the life of the soul is essentially unconscious'[3]; another, that 'the I is first and foremost something bodily.'[4] 'Dance therapy is based on psychoanalytic theory augmented by group dynamics.'[5] In this form of therapy the body is used to express one's own feelings through dancing. Through movement, hidden, unconscious or repressed feelings become conscious and can be expressed. An approach to the unconscious is easier and more directly accessible for some people through dance and drama therapy than through verbal psychotherapy. Severely traumatized people – for instance after physical ill-treatment or sexual abuse – find it difficult to open up in verbal psychotherapy, because the unconscious manipulates their own speech in such a way that the traumatized area remains hidden. The 'experienced body-ego' and the 'real body-ego' are too far apart. These two experiences of the I should converge through dance therapy.

The dancing does not follow any predetermined rules; there is no expectation of an accomplished or aesthetically beautiful performance. The patient is just supposed to move according to the feelings which arise in the moment. Music can be added to the dance. The dancer is not alone; they dance together with others. The others accompany the dancer empathetically, encouraging through careful drumming or singing. In the course of the sessions the patient who previously danced becomes part of this periphery accompanying other fellow-patients.

The process must be guided by an experienced dance therapist, who is psychotherapeutically trained, so that no overreaction arises from the dancer or the helping circle. The therapist must observe how strongly 'constricted' the dancer's movements are and how they relate to the music, the group and to themselves. Their gaze, facial expression, posture, contact with the ground and perception of their surroundings are important criteria in this regard. These can help in assessing the extent to which a patient has resolved their mental or emotional blocks, and how far their experienced body-ego remains separated from their real body-ego. This also determines the number and frequency of their dances.

At the end of each dance, the participants from the circle express what they themselves felt during the dance and what they experienced of the dancer. Through this an intensification of complementary feelings comes about. The dancer learns to observe their experience somewhat from the outside; the circle becomes a mirror and an organ of resonance. The dance may be recorded on video, to enable details subsequently to be examined more closely. Through this secondary observation the dancer can bring the individual elements of expression in their own dance into consciousness and learn to describe it with the therapist.

Ideally the dancer should be able to move freely. However they will be able to express their feelings even if their mobility is restricted; the helping circle will not experience any inability as an essential part of the dance. The flow of movement is not evaluated according to the elements of isotonic or isometric contraction, but solely as to the experience felt. The goal of the therapy is not a functional improvement of the movement system but to become conscious of mental or emotional blockages. Generally the dancer will not know eurythmy's element of feeling. They shape their movements solely out of their feelings and their unconscious desires and hopes. In the process they will alternate unconsciously flowing, oscillating movements, without much development of energy, with contraction, tensing and energetic stillness. Here the trained observer can discover movement and character. The dancer, the surrounding circle and the therapist regard these elements of movement, however, only in respect of their emotional values. These are described in images: 'I experience images of birds, shreds of clouds and of sabres which seem to swish through the air.' 'Social energies' are liberated, which are then put into words as impressions of the dancer, the circle around and the therapist. The aim is to enable integration of the experienced body-ego with the real body-ego.

5.3 Eurythmy therapy between physiotherapy and dance therapy

From the aspect of the three elements movement, feeling and character, and compared with other movement therapies, eurythmy takes its place in the middle.

In physiotherapy objective observation of isotonic and isometric movement exercises predominates. The object of the practice is the mechanically measurable degree of freedom of a movement, or the strength or tone of certain groups of muscles. These are to be improved. The therapy is defined through a somatic conception, and the muscular function restored to health through exercise. Expressed in the language of eurythmy therapy: the therapeutic approach utilizes the elements movement and character, while the feeling element does not consciously resonate along with the others, leaving the therapy's connection to the whole human being incomplete. This therapy may be carried out in groups, although the participants are not reliant on each other in the therapeutic process.

In dance therapy, the dancer expresses unconscious anxieties, inner hindrances or aspirations through the dance movements. The dance may well contain flowing aspects as well as aspects of concentrated force. These formal elements will however be reflected and made conscious only for what they reveal of the feelings. The group is part of the therapeutic journey, the goal of which is to overcome unconscious psychic blocks, repressions and anxieties. These are experienced initially through dancing, then experienced consciously and as far as possible overcome. It is a purely psychotherapeutic approach. In dance therapy, feeling during the dance is given priority.

Eurythmy therapy uses all three elements for its therapeutic task. In the basic eurythmy training the primary sensory experience of movement, feeling and character is developed. These elements are metamorphosed in eurythmy therapy to become effective therapeutically (see Chapter 10).

Eurythmy therapy aspires to activate somatic healing processes through ensouled, experienced movement. This goal will only be attained if the patient experiences anew and enhances their own soul capacities through independent practice. The therapy begins on the functional, etheric level; it unfolds its activity both on the somatic and physiological level and also on the level of soul and spirit. The patient may quite well be introduced to exercises in a group; one-to-one therapy can then indivdualize this.

It is important for the eurythmy therapist to acquire a basic understanding of medicine and psychotherapy. Their own approach, however – both in diagnosis and in therapy – consists in influencing the functions of the ether body. These can be observed in their effects both in the somatic realm and in that of the soul.

One danger should also be mentioned at this point: some eurythmy therapists are fond of using psychological criteria in their movement diagnosis in place of the three elements. This can have a negative influence on the therapeutic approach. The description and evaluation of a movement according to its components of movement, feeling and character are the basis of eurythmy and eurythmy therapy. 'Everything that is to be achieved must be achieved by the eurythmist with movement, feeling and character. Nothing else should come into consideration.'[6]

6. The Consonants

6.1   A classification of consonants

In a conversation among eurythmists, when there is a question about the classification of consonants, the zodiac classification usually comes to mind first. It is in fact documented in a notebook entry as early as 1914;[1] but it is mentioned publicly in a lecture only in 1924:

> Until now our point of departure when characterizing eurythmic gesture has been spoken language ... So today we wish to make an attempt to start from the essential nature of the human being, to seek the forms which can emerge out of the essential nature of the human being ...[2]

Eurythmy had developed up till then solely out of the speaking of sounds.

In 1914, at about the same time as the notebook entry, the 'evolutionary sequence' was given to Tatiana Kisseleff, who wrote: 'Everything that belongs to the evolution of humanity was actually contained [in this evolutionary sequence].'[3]

The classification of consonants in the alphabet should also be mentioned: 'What do you actually do when you utter the alphabet? You immerse yourself to some extent in the form of your ether body and impart it to the air. [As you speak] you form an image of your ether body in the air.'[4] The different classifications of consonants are arranged in Table 2.

The three classifications mentioned so far were not taken as the starting point in the transformation of eurythmy into eurythmy therapy. In the Eurythmy Therapy Course, four other classifications of consonants are described. A first arrangement of the consonants focuses on the spiritual context: in the second lecture *S* is represented as an Ahrimanic sound, *H* as Luciferic and *M* as the consonant in the middle. The difference was said to be observable in the forming of the sounds. This order was not developed further in the subsequent presentation of eurythmy therapy.

The next three sequences of consonants were described in the following lecture; there is one classification which points to a spiritual, inner aspect, alongside a middle sequence and a 'purely external arrangement.'

The Seven Orders of Consonants

1. The zodiac order:
W – R – H – F – D/T – B/P – Ts – S –G/K – L – M – N

The spiritual, shaping forces which work out of macrocosmic space and work in the world timelessly

2. The evolutionary sequence:
B – M – D – N – R – L – G – Ch – F – S – H – T

The shaping forces which have condensed out of the macrocosm enter into time; they are directed toward becoming, toward evolution. A beginning of creation appears.

3. The sequence in the alphabet:
B –C – D – F – G – H – K – L – M – N – P – Q – R – S – T – V – W – Z

The cosmic order changes into an order made by human beings, which appears in writing in the development of culture, but which is not spoken in this order.

4. Ahrimanic and Luciferic Sounds:
S – M – H

All sounds can change their typical form through Ahrimanic or Luciferic impulses. Both forces are active creatively in speech (microcosm) and in all processes of nature.

5. Sounds formed far outside with the vowel after:
K/G – T/D – P/B – W – V – H (German)

When forming these eurythmically, the outside of the arm is emphasized: 'I am far out in the outside world and feel my boundaries with it.'

Sounds formed closer in with the vowel before:
M/N – L – R – F – S – H (English)

When forming these eurythmically, the inside of the arm is emphasized: 'I expand my inner space into my surroundings.'

The unconscious movements of the soul which accompany speech, which become visible in eurythmic formation. In the development of speech, the consonants with the vowel after have lost, in large part, the connection with human movement. The human being, therefore, must go far out of themselves to take hold of these consonants in the world. In the development of speech, this relationship to the human being can be transformed, as with *Phi – eF*.

6. Sounds beginning with:

An impact	(middle sounds)	with blowing
K/G – T/D – P/B	*M/N – L – R*	*F/V/W – Th/S/Sh – Ch*/H*

The sequence of the forming of the consonants in the microcosm of speaking.

Impact sounds begin impactively in speech, ending more blown. Blown sounds begin blowing and end with a delicate impact. Impact sounds begin with the articulation movement, then comes the flow of breath; with the blown sounds, the articulation movement takes hold of the already flowing breath. The middle sounds alternate rhythmically between blowing and impactive components.

7. The location of forming the sound

Palate sounds	*K/G – Ch*/H*	palatal	*R – L – Ng*
Teeth/tongue sound	*T/D – Th/S/Sh*	dental	*R – L – N*
Lip sounds	*P/B – F/V/W*	labial	*R – L – M*

The microcosmic location of the forming of consonants.

Table 2.   * *Ch* as in Scottish 'loch'

The Eurythmy Therapy Course is based on these three classifications. The first sequence (the fifth classification in Table 2) is based on the way in which the vowel is brought in when speaking a consonant. The vowel can be placed after, as with *Ha*, or before, as with *eF*. The transformation of the ancient Greek *Phi*, with the vowel after, to the *eF* of today was an important phenomenon in the development of humanity's soul-awareness. When the vowel is placed after as in *Ha*, the human being is concerned to seek 'the spiritual, through speech, in the outer object; when they speak an *eF*, they are more concerned to relate to the spiritual within.' Whether the onset of the forming of a sound still comes wholly from the periphery, or whether the human being has already separated from an experience of the periphery, and the onset onset of forming a consonant is closer to their own body, should be expressed visually when an individual consonant is being shown in eurythmy.

The second classification (the sixth classification in Table 2) relates to the movement of the consonants. The dynamic of the stream of air, in damming-up and moving, is examined and then metamorphosed into eurythmy (as well as into eurythmy therapy). The polarity of the impact and blown sounds is developed, and the following said: 'In relation to the attributes I am now speaking about, eurythmy has to proceed in a way polar opposite to that of the actual process of speaking.' *H* is given as an extreme blown sound, *B* as an obvious impact sound; later the sounds *R* and *L* as mediating between the two extremes.

The polar speech movement of blown and impact sounds is examined more closely in order to form a foundation for the transformation of speech movement into eurythmy movement. The sound movement in the speaking of impact sounds begins with the impact, which gives these sounds their name. The stream of air is first dammed up by a narrowing made by the tongue or the lips in the region of the palate or the teeth. The sound-specific occlusion is brought in before the air flows on in the outbreath. The occlusion is then suddenly opened. The air can now stream out, formed by the speech instrument, and the impact sound is uttered.

The process with blown sounds is the opposite. With these, utterance begins when the air which is already moving is shaped through the positioning of the speech instrument. The forming and the streaming of the air are simultaneous and not consecutive as with the impact sounds. At the same time, the onset of the blown sounds need a gentle glottal push. This initial sound (aleph) arises beyond the place where the palatal sounds are formed, near the larynx. The same initial sound is also formed at the beginning of speaking vowels. It is the same for all blown sounds and vowels and belongs to the realm of sounds that were uttered before speech was articulated. It is a precondition for, but not part of, a blown sound.

The actual speaking begins with the forming of the blowing, streaming, oscillating air. At the end, the flowing movement when speaking an *H*, an *S* or an *F* is rounded off with a slight impact, brought about by arresting the stream of air. Without such a slight impacting conclusion, one would no longer be speaking but just exhaling strongly.

In summarizing, the following can be said: in speech, the impact sounds begin with the impact and end more with blowing; the blown sounds begin with blowing and flowing, only to end with a barely perceived impact. At the same time both groups may be spoken hard, as with *K* or *Ch* (as in lo*ch*, not *ch*eese), or more softly, as with *G* or *H*. The middle sounds are characterized by the way the blowing and impacting elements in the formation of the sound follow each other rapidly. They do not begin or finish with a clear-cut impact or blowing; in the course of speech both aspects of the movement alternate.

The 'purely external' arrangement of the consonants (7th classification in Table 2) looks at the location where these are formed. Impact sounds can be formed on the palate (*K*, *G*), more on the teeth (*T*, *D*) or on the lips (*P*, *B*). The blown sounds, too, divide into lip sounds (*W*, *F*, *V*), teeth sounds (*Sh*, *S*, *Ts*) and palate (soft palate) sounds (*H*, *Ch*).

What is clear is that the last three of the classifications described arise wholly out of the speaking human being and not from a cosmic perspective.

In the Eurythmy Therapy Course, the movement classification of speech is presented most extensively. For that reason it should be studied first quite closely. The impact and blown sounds (and the vibrating and wave sounds between them) may be arranged schematically in such a way that the most impactive sounds and the most blown sound are looked at as polar opposites. In this way the classification presented in Figure 2 arises.

With the impact sounds, the sound formation goes from the palatal sounds *K* and *G*, via the teeth [dental] sounds *T* and *D*, until it comes to the lip [labial] sounds *P* and *B*. On this journey, the 'impactiveness' of the sound steadily declines. For the blown sounds, the place of onset of speech also moves in the mouth from palate to lips. The same decline in degree of blowing also takes place: the *H* arises on the soft palate, the *Ch* distinctly further forward. The *Sh*, and more decidedly the *S*, *Z* and *Ts*, have their onset at the teeth; while *F*, *V* and *W* are formed with the lips.

The sounds which lie between the two poles are here called middle sounds. They have in common that they can sound in the different regions of the speech organs; in certain dialects the palate *R* or soft-palate *R* predominates, in others the tongue *R*. A similar flexibility also applies to the *L*. In German, it is a teeth sound; in English, on the other hand, a soft

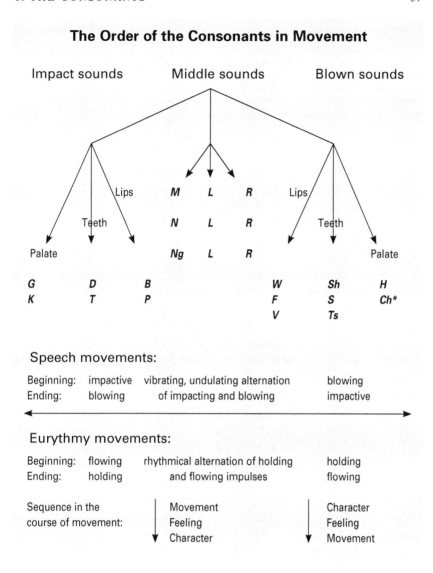

The Order of the Consonants in Movement

Impact sounds   Middle sounds   Blown sounds

	Lips	M	L	R	Lips		
Teeth		N	L	R		Teeth	
Palate		Ng	L	R			Palate

G	D	B			W	Sh	H
K	T	P			F	S	Ch*
					V	Ts	

Speech movements:

| Beginning: | impactive | vibrating, undulating alternation | blowing |
| Ending: | blowing | of impacting and blowing | impactive |

Eurythmy movements:

| Beginning: | flowing | rhythmical alternation of holding | holding |
| Ending: | holding | and flowing impulses | flowing |

| Sequence in the course of movement: | Movement Feeling Character | Character Feeling Movement |

Figure 2. The sequence of consonants arranged according to their speech movements and eurythmy movements.

palate sound. For little children, the speaking of consonants begins with a sound which resembles a lip *R* or lip *L* or *M*. These lip sounds are initially hardly distinguishable from each other. The place where these middle sounds are formed alters, but not the kind of movement while sounding. From the point of view that the forming of the sound for the same consonant is possible at different places within the mouth, *M*, *N* and the nasal sound *Ng* form a direct transition from the impact to the middle sounds.

The lip sound *M*, the teeth sound *N* further in, and the nasal sound *Ng* on the soft palate arise through the change of location, like *R* and *L*. In speaking the *M*, *N* or nasal *Ng*, the flow of air is comparable.

At this point, the suggested classification diverges from those mentioned in the fourth lecture of the Eurythmy Therapy Course and also in the speech and drama course. In line with normal usage it is said there that *M* and *N* are the softest impact sounds. In the classification used here *M* and *N* appear as transitions; they are the 'most impactive' middle sounds. The frequently utilized allocation of impact and blown sounds to the four elements comes only in the Speech and Drama Course.[5] Many physicians prescribe consonants as a therapeutic medium according to their elemental category: the blown sounds correlate with the element of fire; the impact sounds, including *M* and *N*, with the element of earth. *L* is the water sound and *R* that of air.

Concerning the eurythmic forming of the consonants as blown, middle and impact sounds, the following is stated in the course as a principle: 'since – in respect to the characteristic of which I am thinking at the moment – the eurythmical element has to stand as polar opposite to the actual process in speech' (p. 32). Speech movement and eurythmy movement must be polar opposite to each other. This immediately becomes clear from the following. The impact sounds in speech all begin with the impactive part and end in blowing. Polar to that, the eurythmic movements begin flowing and streaming and end in a final conformation that has an impactive, contracting character. The following applies to the eurythmic forming of all the impact sounds: a streaming start to the movement, ending in a fixed final form. The blown sounds are shaped in the polar opposite way: the eurythmic movements begin with a drawn-together, held starting position and end more or less flowing outward. The gesture of speech is again the opposite; the uttering of these sounds begins blowing and ends with a slight impact. This relationship is illustrated in Figure 2.

6.2   A classification of eurythmy therapy indications for the consonants

The classification in Figure 2 of the movements in the spoken consonants may be viewed as a natural arrangement. It proves its value when the eurythmy therapy indications mentioned in the course are brought together with this natural order. The speech-oriented classification and the conceptual sequence of the indications back each other up, indicating a congruence.

The indications as to how individual consonants work in the metabolism are described in the fourth lecture. We shall relate these therapeutic indications to the previously developed classification according to speech. An astonishing symmetry arises.

The enumeration of these indications starts with the two extreme impact and blown sounds (Figure 3) overleaf.

6.2.1 Indications for palate sounds

The *K* and *G* movements 'stimulate the onward motion, the inner mechanization of the intestine, and thus promote the movement of the intestine itself' (p. 48).

The *H* movement has a strong effect on the regulation of intestinal activity in the area of transition from the stomach into the intestine ... if someone cannot get their food from the stomach into the intestine' (p.51). The sound tends to be used in cases of pylorospasm.

These sounds work – in different places – on the mechanical muscle activity of the gastrointestinal tract. The intention is to promote peristaltic movement. This results in both places from the regulated alternation of tightening and letting go. The spatial movement forward of the content, the chyme or the faeces, enabled by the activity of the muscle, is disturbed in both cases and is normalized through the polar palate sound. In Figure 3 the indications are charted in order to facilitate an overview.

K, G and *H* have a regulating effect on the muscular activity in the gastrointestinal tract.

6.2.2 Indications for the teeth sounds

The difference is emphasized between *G* and *K*, which have already been described, and *D* and *T*, where 'the processing of the food itself is more affected, while with *G, K* and *Q* the effect is more on the onward motion of foods in the intestine.' The *D* and *T* movements work 'to strengthen the intestinal activity, particularly when that activity manifests itself in constipation. In this manner one can counteract constipation in many cases.' (p. 48).

The *S* movement is applied for adults and children '... who show insufficient digestive activity and who consequently have headaches, since this movement regulates in particular the formation of gas in the intestine' (p. 49).

The *Sh* movement, as the softer middle blown sound, 'affects the beginning portions of the intestinal tract that pertain to the stomach.' And where 'stomach acidity easily occurs and so on' (p. 54).

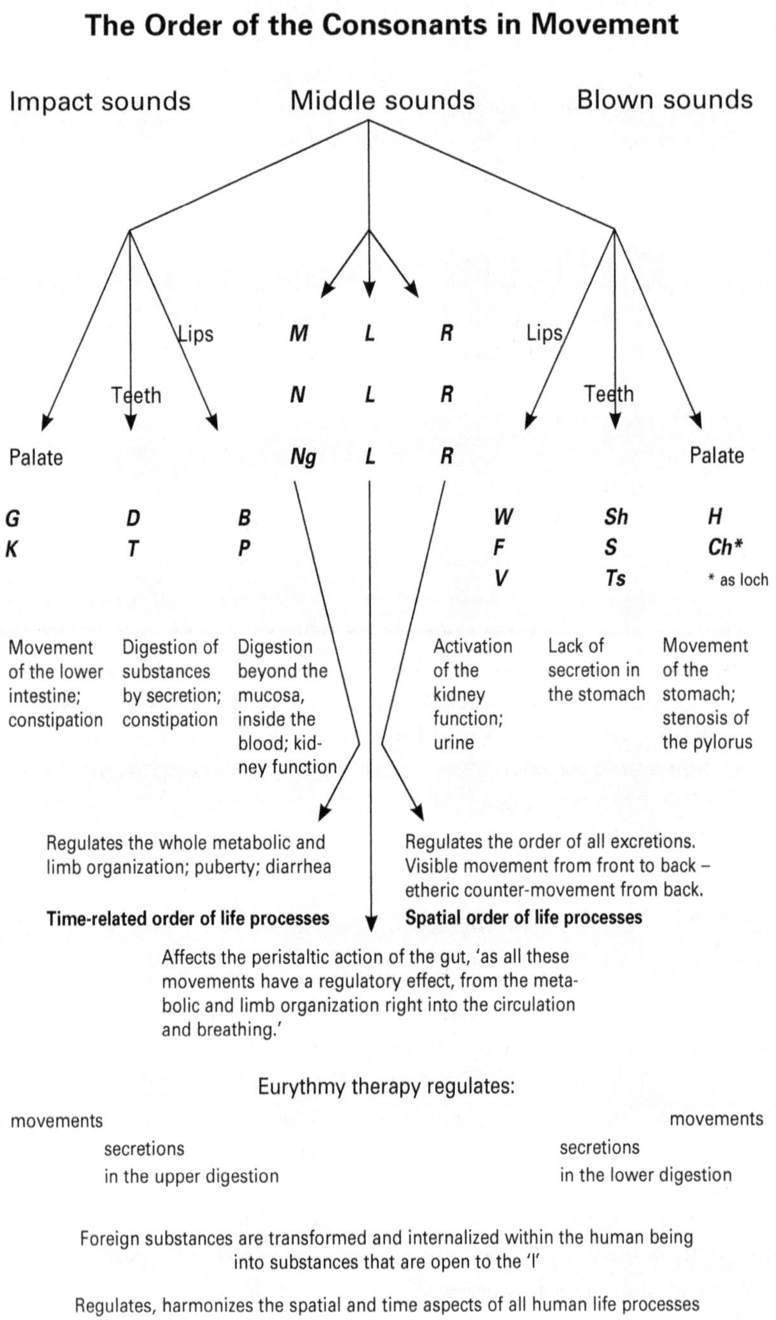

The Order of the Consonants in Movement

Impact sounds   Middle sounds   Blown sounds

Lips   **M**   **L**   **R**   Lips

Teeth   **N**   **L**   **R**   Teeth

Palate   **Ng**   **L**   **R**   Palate

G	**D**	**B**		**W**	**Sh**	**H**
K	**T**	**P**		**F**	**S**	**Ch***
				V	**Ts**	* as loch

Movement of the lower intestine; constipation	Digestion of substances by secretion; constipation	Digestion beyond the mucosa, inside the blood; kidney function	Activation of the kidney function; urine	Lack of secretion in the stomach	Movement of the stomach; stenosis of the pylorus

Regulates the whole metabolic and limb organization; puberty; diarrhea

Time-related order of life processes

Regulates the order of all excretions. Visible movement from front to back – etheric counter-movement from back.

Spatial order of life processes

Affects the peristaltic action of the gut, 'as all these movements have a regulatory effect, from the metabolic and limb organization right into the circulation and breathing.'

Eurythmy therapy regulates:

movements   movements

secretions   secretions

in the upper digestion   in the lower digestion

Foreign substances are transformed and internalized within the human being into substances that are open to the 'I'

Regulates, harmonizes the spatial and time aspects of all human life processes

Figure 3. Correlation of the eurythmy therapy indications with the speech sequence of consonants.

The kind of constipation which is treated through *T* is attributable to insufficient elimination of digestive secretions and intestinal mucus. The disorder which is described in connection with *S*, associated with gas formation and headaches, is treated with bitter remedies as its medication. The elimination of digestive secretions in the region of the gall bladder and the pancreas is thereby stimulated. The *S* strengthens the same function; for *Sh*, the soft sound, stomach acidity 'and so on' are mentioned as the target of the therapy.

T and *D*, *S* and *Sh* work on the glandular secretions into the gastrointestinal tract. Through these secretions, the foreign nature of food can be overcome. They are the precondition for healthy ingestion of food.

With both the teeth and the palate sounds, a difference between impact and blown sound is indicated. The effects of the blown sounds, that is of the *H* and the *S*, should have their onset in the stomach and upper intestine. The place of efficacy of the impact sounds is located further below, in the large intestine. These are the only indications for the different effects of impact and blown sounds.

6.2.3   *Indications for the lip sounds*

B and *P* 'work back on the inward digestion, on all that is digestive activity in the blood vessels, and in particular on what is digestive activity in the kidneys. So if you are concerned with regulating activity of the kidneys, you would have such movements carried out.' (p. 47).

The *F* movement 'has a stimulating effect on the passing of urine.' No further indication is given as to what kind of renal or bladder disorder is concerned. *V* (German *W*), the soft, blown lip sound, is not mentioned in the Course.

The two lip sounds *B* and *F* have in common that in each case the renal and urinary tract is mentioned. The physiological correlative for *B* is fortunately described clearly: beyond the intestinal wall, in the blood, in connection with the kidneys.

The sequence of indications leads from the simple movements of the muscles in the gut (*K* and *H*), to the secretions which are released into the interior of the intestine and which enable the initial processing of food (*T* and *S*, *Sh*). If the path taken by food as it is processed in the organism is followed further, it is necessary to examine the passage of the broken-down foodstuffs from the bowel into the blood and how individualized substances are built up. This physiologically necessary step is also followed in the sequence of indications for the lip sounds. The transition of substances through the wall of the bowel and into the blood is given as an indication for *B*.

The place of the kidneys in this transformation of nutrition (beyond the intestinal wall) is described in detail by Steiner in a general lecture and shortly after in a medical lecture.[6] The content of these lectures will be reviewed briefly in order better to substantiate the therapeutic potential of the lip sounds.

In the intestine, the chyme consists of substances which still contain much of their original vitality. This is still the case if the original state has been altered through cooking and other preparation. For a long time this mush of foodstuffs still displays properties which point to the vitality of the foods. The specific traces of vitality must be broken down and completely destroyed in the upper gastrointestinal tract. The mush of nutrients has to become both 'mineral and liquid.' This mineralizing is the precondition for all the following stages. In both lectures it is described how, afterward, the stream of substances is carried over the boundary of the intestine and into the blood. The mineral, fluid substance is re-enlivened thereby. This transformation takes place in a field of forces which develops between the heart and the lung. Those substances which cannot be re-enlivened are eliminated though the intestine or exhaled. After that, the organism guides the stream of substances which are already within the blood into another field of forces. This second field extends between the brain and the kidneys. Here the substances are transformed further, gaining a new capacity, becoming carriers of soul qualities. The parts of substance which cannot sufficiently be lifted to this stage are excreted through the kidney in the urine.

Finally, the initially foreign substances are further transformed: in the field of forces between sense organs and liver they attain their relation to the I, their openness for the I. Substances which have not yet attained the qualitative enhancement to this capacity for the I are excreted with the gall and only taken up again later. This qualitative metamorphosis of substances from a mineral quality to one capable of carrying the I is thereby completed. These substances are now able to build up an individual human body. Up to that point they had not been specialized for the different organs, but can now be used by the I for building up all the organs. In the sixth medical lecture of the course held parallel to the Eurythmy Therapy Course, this ascending stream of substance which takes its course in the blood is described as the 'unstable protein organization ... In the tissue fluid a continual assimilation and destruction of the protein contained in food takes place.'[7]

The sequence of transformation of substances cited here is a result of spiritual research. It will still be necessary to work out in more detail which physiological correlates are meant when the fields of force 'heart and lung,' 'brain and kidney' and 'sense organs and liver' are mentioned.

In the eurythmy therapy lecture only two partial areas of this meta-morphosis of substance are mentioned: 'beyond the intestinal wall' and 'kidney.' But there is no doubt that the same sequence of transformation is meant. It begins from the intestine and guides the stream of substances through the blood and into the areas where processes of lung, kidney and liver are at work. This series of processes is indicated by the following: *B* and *P* 'work back on the inward digestion, on all that is digestive activity in the blood vessels, and in particular on what is digestive activity in the kidneys. So if you are concerned with regulating activity of the kidneys, you would have such movements carried out.' (p. 47).

Based on the inner symmetry of the whole sequence it may be assumed that this thought is also valid for the blown lip sound *F*. In the lecture only the urine formation is mentioned in connection with *F*. But there is no doubt that the indication for *F* is a part of the series mentioned in full above. Which disorder of urine formation or urination is meant is not clear from the text. A difference between the effect of impact and blown sound is also left open in the text.

B, *P* and *F* effect the transition of substances from a foreign, min-eral quality to one which is open to the self, the I. This condition of substance informed by the I is described elsewhere as pure warmth.[8] The substances do not as yet bear the imprint of a particular organ. A material informed by the I has come into being which is available to every process of building up in the organism. The I-enabled substance can be used for building bones or for the regeneration of the liver or the brain. However the I-character of the organism must always be maintained; the ether body has to implement the processes of building up step-by-step.

6.2.4 Indications for the middle sounds

Lastly, the middle sounds will be looked at. The sound that stands right in the middle of the sequence will be considered first. The *L* movement stimulates the organism, from intestinal peristalsis, from the 'system of the limbs and the metabolism into what ... is ... adjacent to it, that is into the circulation and into the respiratory movement as well' (p. 50). With the therapeutic indications up to this point, the target for their effect lay in the realm of the substances connected with nutrition: from the movement of the chyme in the bowel, via the breaking down of foreign foodstuffs through secretions, right up to the metamorphosis into individualized substances. With the *L*-movement, the building up goes far beyond these areas of function: right into the circulation and the breathing.

The *R* is described in quite a different style:

It is particularly interesting to see how the movement, which as a movement of the intestine progresses from the front to the back, releases a movement in the etheric body which proceeds from back to front and then breaks on the abdominal wall, ... disappears ... This activity which counters the physical movement will be aroused, for example, particularly by the *R*-movement. (p. 56)

Compared to the previous descriptions, the observable symptom withdraws; a counter-process is emphasized. Connected with this is the fact that all discernible movements of the inner organs and the limbs always have their counter-processes. Unnoticed compensating counter-movements take place everywhere. These unobserved elements are called 'etheric.' Through the *R*, it is not the movements themselves (as with *K* and *H*) but the inner, unobserved counter movements and processes that are activated, in order to build up of the organism. One may suppose that the *R* generally improves the organism's ability to balance movement and counter-movement. The text of the lecture is again open to narrow or broader interpretation.

At this point the *M* should be mentioned as a transition from the impact to the middle sounds, together with the harder *N* and the nasal *Ng*. We pointed out earlier that these sounds are formed with the same speech movement in different places. At the same time it is assumed that *M* and *N* as softer and harder sounds have a similar indication.

The indication for the *M*-movement is special, as it is the only one to have a reference to development of the organism over time. *M* 'acts to regulate the entire system of the metabolism and the limbs. It is extraordinarily important to practise it with with children during puberty' (p. 51). Maria Glas writes about this: 'In the first place, *M* was given for children in adolescence who were in some way overwhelmed by the onslaught of new drives and feelings. The essence of this malady is that the ordering forces are not able to meet this onslaught from below.'[9] 'During puberty,' or literally, the 'age of children's development' is, of course, more than just puberty with its specific issues. The effect of the *M* movement emphasizes the possibility to influence the chronological organization of building up processes. Compared with the *R*, where the spatial aspect was emphasized in the course, the indication here relates to chronological ordering of an etheric process.

N is mentioned before and after the description of gymnastics. The *N* movement 'greatly strengthens the intestinal activity, and in such a manner that it can be applied where there is a tendency to diarrhea' (p. 52). Again, just the symptom is mentioned, not the underlying disorder. On the morning of the same day, Steiner describes diarrhea in detail in the medical lecture: the upper forces are meant to break down foreign nutriment. A lack of these forces leads to the substances remaining too strongly foreign and vital; symptoms of diarrhea thereby arise, which can lead to breakdown of the mucous membrane of the intestine. A predominance of the lower processes leads to the disintegration of the individual's own organ structure. The upper forces, (here also called arsenizing forces) are to be intensified by the remedy of arsenic. Through this, the foreign life of the substances can be destroyed and the diarrhea stopped. When the two descriptions from the Eurythmy Therapy Course and the Medical Course are taken together the following process becomes apparent: the foreign quality of the nourishment is not sufficiently eradicated. The upper forces are too weak and the symptom of diarrhea appears through the dominance of the lower forces. Arsenic strengthens the upper forces establishing the balance, but cannot of itself heal the damage inside the intestine. The actual healing process of the organ has to be activated by other remedies or through the *N*, which calls on the building up lower human being as counter-process to the arsenic.

Again it is possible to observe a process in time, as with the *M*: the therapeutic aim is not directed at the illness itself; rather at regulating a process resulting from the illness. The initial therapy is the arsenic; the actual healing is stimulated through the subsequent counter-process. The text from the course gives no indication for a process in time influenced by the *N*. However the whole picture, once organized and arranged, calls for this amplification: the *N* is indicated whenever previous therapeutic measures run the risk of setting off over-reactions. The *N*-movement regulates the successive phases of therapy.

6.3 Summary

The consonants are organized in a comprehensible sequence between blowing and impacting. They all work within the metabolism in an building-ing up way. This is summarized in Figure 3.

1. The palate sounds *K, G* and *H* activate the movement of the intestinal tract.
2. The teeth sounds *T, D* and *S, Sh* activate the preparation of digestive secretions in the whole digestive tract. They are essential aids to overcoming the foreignness of food.
3. The lip sounds *P, B* and *F* activate those forces in the organism which gradually refine substances from mineral nature into the quality of the self, the I. The substance which finally arises can carry the I, but is still undifferentiated. It can be transformed into any specialized organ substance. It can be used for building blood or bone, liver tissue or

nerve tissue. This specialization of universal substance is achieved in the next step.

4. The force which enables the building up of individual organs out of the universally human substance which is capable of bearing the self, the I, is stimulated through the transitional middle sounds *M, N* and *L* and *R*. One can take as an example for this the healing of a broken bone. The ether body has to have the force to actuate the building up of bone at the place where it is injured, not just in the bone system generally. This spatial aspect is emphasized when it comes to the *R*. In addition, the ether body has to direct the sequence of healing. Both the breaking down of the damaged bone-substance and the building up of the new callus occur in a regulated sequence. This chronological aspect is emphasized with the *M*; while for the *N* the sequence of the different phases of therapy is indicated. With the *L*, as the central consonant, all the building up processes of the ether body are orchestrated: the building up of blood and bones, the healing of nerves and sense organs, and regeneration everywhere.

6.4   The work of blown and impact sounds in the organism

Differentiation of the blown and impact sounds, when observed in their speech movement and their eurythmy gesture, is easy. The sequence of the blown and impactive elements in speech can be clearly recognized. The progression of movement and character elements of both groups of sounds in eurythmy also reveals a polar placement. In contrast to this obvious polarity, the different indications for the blown and impact sounds are not straightforward. In the description of the individual sounds, it has already been indicated that the impact sounds *K* and *G* are applied for movement disorders in the region of the lower intestine; while for the blown sound *H* it is the stomach area. In the same way, the impact sounds *T* and *D* are indicated for disorders involving the secretions in the large intestine; the blown sounds *S* and *Sh* for those in the stomach and duodenum. These two places are the only pointers in the Eurythmy Therapy Course to how the indications for impact and blown sounds can be differentiated.

So we can carefully generalize once more: the impact sounds appear to work lower down in the body than the blown sounds. The building up process in the human body requires different qualities, depending on whether the nutritional stream is observed in the sensory-nerve system or in the metabolism. The sense organs and the brain need a different quality of substance for maintenance and growth to that needed by the muscles, and so on. All consonants affect the stream of building up forces: the blown sounds appear to promote building up in the head and breathing system; the impact sounds promote it in the lower body.

It is then possible to generalize as follows:

1. Forces of movement are promoted
— in the metabolism through the impact sounds K and G
— in the nerve-sense and breathing systems through the blown sound H

2. The building up of secretions and substances used for specialized processes are promoted
— in the metabolism and circulatory systems through the impact sounds T and D
— in the nerve-sense and breathing systems through the blown sounds S and Sh

3. The building up of the individual's own substance is promoted
— up to the point where it has the capacity to bear qualities of the etheric and of the soul, through the impact sounds P and B
— up to the point where it can assimilate the self, the I, through the blown sound F

4. The building up of the substances of organs is regulated
— spatially through the R
— chronologically through N and M
— L stands in the centre of all building up life processes, integrating all building up in the organism, and orchestrating the source-point of all becoming.

The working of all consonants must have a correspondence with all the building up processes in the human organism. This entirety of the building up processes can be seen in the Eurythmy Therapy Course only if one does not read the text literally, but takes the individual indications as examples of a specialized area of the metabolism. The classification of the consonants presented here refers to the entirety of building up processes in the organism. The classification arises on the one hand from the order of speaking, on the other from the order of building up processes enabled in transforming food. The entirety of building up processes in the organism comprises the individual life-processes of maintenance, growth and reproduction.[10] The physiological functions of these life-processes are described elsewhere.[11]

7. The Vowels

7.1 Classifications of the vowels in Rudolf Steiner's work

The well-known vowel order *A, E, I, O, U* appears in a number of different lectures by Rudolf Steiner. The significance of the sequence is underlined in the statement: 'If one just lets the five vowels work on one in succession, one gains the impression of a fresh, pristine human being. The human being gives birth to himself again in full worth when he lets these five vowels sound forth in full consciousness.'[1] In the Creative Speech Course, the sequence of vowels was also built up in this order:

Consider the *A*. A child can do it: one opens the mouth wide and sends the stream of speech through; the child enjoys doing that. *A* is the least configured; with *U* on the other hand you have to purse your lips, not just shape them plastically, but configure them to the greatest extent. The other vowels are in between. If you modify the simple procedure that you have with *A*, draw it together more, you get *E*; draw together even more: *I*; and if you enlist the aid of your lips and make a circle of them: *O*. You don't need to purse your lips for that yet, only when you come to *U*.[2]

This standard sequence is also in the forefront of the therapy recommendations in the works of Bort, Kirchner-Bockholt and Glas.

It is all the more striking when a different order of the vowels is used in particular places. The one concerned is the vowel sequence *A, E, O, U, I* or, the other way round, *I, U, O, E, A*. In the lectures on education the following statement is made, 'The child normally acquires the vowels in this sequence ... *A – E – O – U – I*.'[3] A different statement is found in a note in connection with an esoteric exercise for attaining inner quiet: '*I, U, O, E, A*. The vowels in this sequence must only inwardly be brought to intonation, so that they gain more and more forces and, in creating, fill the physical ear from within to without – Christ speaks.'[4] The inward, meditative intoning of the vowel sequence allows inner quiet to arise and furthers the spiritual development of the human being.

On the one hand, the normal sequence *A, E, I, O, U* appears to correspond to the spatial, physical succession of sound formation from the soft palate *A* to the lip *U*; on the other, it arises out of the soul's feelings. In the marvelling *A*, childlike sympathy streams into the world. In *E* the forces appear which close off and repel, which enable an experience of self. In the sound *I*, the human being returns to a unity with the world now intended out of freedom; in *O*, the human being feels themself as a soul. In *U* fear and longing for further development appear.[5] The significance of this sequence of sounds, and the moods of soul which belong to them, are also described at length by Barfod.[6]

The unaccustomed sequence *A, E, O, U, I* points to something different. With the normal sequence, the locality of the sound formation and the soul's resonance can be experienced. However, in this sequence, a living process appears. It shows the acquisition of speech during the development of the child, as well as the gradual attainment of a higher consciousness. This 'living' sequence also appears when we look at the movements while uttering of the vowels. *A*, as the most primal vowel, can be transformed with a rounded tongue, on the one hand, into *O* and *U*; with a straight tongue, on the other, into *E* and *I* (Figures 4a and 4b).

The description in the Eurythmy Therapy Course ties in with these vowel sequences: the unfamiliar sequence (in reverse order) *I, U, O, E, A* appears twice in the second lecture, first in the sequence used to introduce the vowels then when they are summarized, 'The *I* [*ee*] reveals the human being as a person; the *U* reveals the human as human being; the *O* reveals the human being as soul; the *E* fixes the self, the ego in the etheric body, ... the *A* counteracts the animal-nature in the human being' (pp. 21f). In this enumeration, all the vowels work on the human being's different constituent entities: the *U* on the human being as human being (consciousness soul); the sound *I* as person (mind soul); the *O* as sentient soul; the *E* on the ether body. Only *A* is described with another category. What is meant here? ('The *A* counteracts the animal nature in the human being.') The *A* occupies a special position; at another point it was emphasized for the eurythmists: '*A* is the human being in greatest perfection.'[7] The *A* relates to a development taking place in a living body, beginning in mineral, physical existence, which overcomes that condition and develops itself further into the realm of the living and the animal or astral, in order to ascend to the height of the human self – 'the human being in their greatest perfection.'

A further relation is shown by the indications: the *I* and *U* are mentioned together for a problem with walking and standing; *O* and *E* are described as having polar effects on fatness and thinness. The *A* stands alone; it has no partner. This vowel sequence, *I–U, O–E* and *A*, beside its special significance for living developmental processes, has

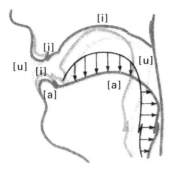
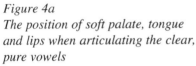
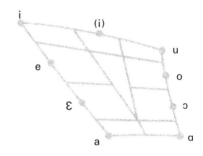

Figure 4a
The position of soft palate, tongue
and lips when articulating the clear,
pure vowels

Figure 4b
Diagram of the locations where
vowels are formed in the vowel
rectangle

After Pompino-Marschall, © Copyright by Walter de Gruyter 1995

a cognitive task for therapy. The diphthongs appear if the vowels are pronounced in the order which Steiner is using here: *A–O–U* forms the *Au* and *A–E–I* the *Ei*. Neither is mentioned in the Eurythmy Therapy Course.

7.2   The relation of speech and eurythmy to the vowels

The eurythmic forming of the consonants arises out of the law of polarity: the gestures in eurythmy are polar to those when speaking the sounds aloud. This is shown clearly in the Eurythmy Therapy Course, and was described in Chapter 6. As far as the vowels are concerned, a similar connection between the flow of speech and the eurythmy movements has so far received little attention. In order to gather material for this question, the speech movement of the vowels will first be examined in some detail.

The normal sequence of vowel sounds from *A* through *E, I* and *O* to *U* will be used for that. The following explanations use descriptions from *Introduction to Phonetics* by Pompino-Marschall and from *Lehrbuch der Phoniatrie und Pädaudiologie* by Wendler, Seidner and Eysholt.

The pure vowels are clearly recognizable in the German language; in many other languages they are combined into diphthongs. During speech, the vowels arise from the oscillations which come into being in the air within the speech instrument. Only this oscillating is not fixed, as in an organ pipe, because the shape and size of the space in which the oscillation takes place is variable in many different ways. The speech instrument between larynx and lips is formed anew for each vowel. Put very simply, two spaces can be distinguished: the speech instrument between the larynx and the roof of the throat; and the horizontal element between the uvula at the back, and the lips (Figure 4a). In these two spaces, the air resonates at certain frequencies called formants. In the diagrams in Figures 5a and 5b, the two formants and their frequencies for the pure vowels are given.

The A sounds when the lowest space in the throat is fully closed and the speech instrument in front of that is widely opened through the tongue's being kept low. The A is thus the most open vowel. The open A (as in 'bard') comes about the furthest back; the shorter A (as in 'bud') is formed somewhat further forward. Between the entirely open A and the entirely closed A there are transitions (Figure 4b, lower horizontal line). This simple intoning of the A can be modified in two different directions.

First, to form the I sound (as in 'bee'), the lower space within the throat, which was narrowed for the A, is opened and the tongue is raised toward the forward palate; the tongue reaches its highest position and narrows the resonance space at the roof of the throat. Along the middle of the tongue a valley is formed and on each side a little mound appears. At the same time, the space of the mouth is marginally lengthened through the position of the lips. The vowel E (the closest English equivalent is 'bake') arises through a position which lies between A and I: the sounding space between the constriction at the palate and the lips is somewhat longer and more open than with the I. The central valley is less pronounced, and several smaller mounds appear on each side. The tongue stays unrounded for both sounds.

Secondly, when the U (as in 'moo') is spoken, the lower space of the throat remains wide open, as with the I. The tongue is positioned quite high and far back, rounded at the sides, and the lips are rounded and pursed. The constriction now lies, on the one hand, at the back of the roof of the throat, on the other hand, right at the front. A lengthened resonance chamber now arises in both the vertical and horizontal parts. Through the enlarging of the resonance space, the frequency of both formants is reduced to a low level. U is the most closed vowel. For O (as in 'ocean'), the tongue is also rounded, the resonance distances somewhat shorter, and the frequencies of both formants also somewhat higher than with U.

The three vowels A, I and U are also referred to as 'corner vowels.' The other pure vowels E and O, and all their nuances, arise as intermediary positions between the corner vowels, as can be seen in the diagrams (Figures 4 & 5).

From the speech movement of the vowels, a first transformation series arises on the basis of the A, via the E to the I; a second series via the O to the corner vowel U.

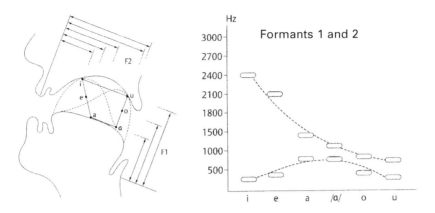

Figure 5a and 5b (after Wendler). The vowel rectangle, which shows diagrammatically the position of the first and second formants in relation to the articulatory position of the tongue.

The process forming the speech organs during embryonic development determines the location where the vowels are uttered. There is a similar process in eurythmy therapy: the *A* stands alone, providing a foundation on which a first duality of *O* and *E*, and a further one of *U* and *I*, can be established. This similarity of the vowel formation in the speech instrument with the arrangement of vowels in the therapeutic indications does not, however, answer the question as to how the eurythmic vowels relate to speech.

The beginnings of a possible arrangement are to be found in the third lecture of the Eurythmy Therapy Course in the description of *U* and *O*:

[*U*] is the sound which in a certain respect expresses its physiological-pathological connection even in the manner in which it is formed in speech. The *U* is spoken with the mouth and the openings between the teeth constricted to the greatest degree and with the lips somewhat extended ... You can see that in speaking one seeks an essentially outward movement with the *U*. In the pronunciation of *U* the to characterize something moving predominates. Thus with the eurythmical *U*, the physiologic opposite occurs: the ability to stand firm is called forth. This is present in the *U* in artistic eurythmy as well, at least as a suggestion.

If you now take a look at the other vowels you will find a progressive internalization. In the case of the *O* you have the lips pushed together towards the front and the opening of the mouth reduced in size ... This is transformed into the polar opposite in the encompassing gesture of the *O*-movement in eurythmy. (p. 37).

Unfortunately, Steiner describes here only the pronunciation of *U* and *O*, without describing the other vowels.

It is clear from the passage quoted that there is also a polar relation between the movement of the vowels in speech and their formation in eurythmy. The speaking of the *U* took place furthest toward the outside; there was the greatest mobility here (with the lowest frequencies). In the following sentence the therapeutic aim for the eurythmy movement of the *U* is mentioned, but the transformation of speech movement into that of eurythmy is not described. The *O* is less closed when speaking than the *U* and is less far toward the outside – how can something 'all-encompassing' arise from it? Nor is the transformation of the speech movement into eurythmy mentioned with the other sequence (*E* and *I*).

In another series of lectures the statement is made: '*E* appears to us in such a way that if we actually take the exhaled air as a model in the [eurythmic] *E* movement, something can arise for us as an imagination like streams crossing each other.'[8] The crossing that characterizes the eurythmy *E* is perceptible imaginatively in speech. But how does the crossing manifest in the physiology of speech? It must remain open as to which element of movement in speech correlates with the crossing in the eurythmy *E*.

After this brief indication as to how the movements of the vowels in speech and eurythmy are related, the description in the third lecture of the Eurythmy Therapy Course changes to a new theme. The formative working of *O* and *E*, which is active before birth, is presented: one should consider the development of form in the human being. 'The forces which are present in the upper human being and which tend toward expansion' are activated through the *O* as a cosmic sound. This formative force is connected with the whole development of the cosmos. During embryonic development, this *O* force leads to the early growth of the brain and to broadening in the formation of the skull, to a rounding of the head. After the infant stage, it is no longer able to work in this place, also because of the closed sutures. If it is stimulated through a speech that is rich in *O*, the *O* then continues this gesture in the region of the torso. The tendency to obesity arises. The organism can become broadened out, thickened, in the surrounding layer of fat.

In a polar fashion the *E*, as a cosmic formation, activates 'the forces which are present in the lower human being and which have a tendency toward the linear ... What manifests with the *E* is that human beings [during their embryonic development] want to take hold of themselves, pull themselves together inwardly.' The outcome of this tendency leads before birth to the crossing of the nerves from the right side to the left and vice versa. This 'pulling together' also manifests in the uniting of the motor and sensory nerves in the forebrain and spinal ganglion, and in the synaptic networking of the brain with the spinal cord and the whole torso. In embryonic development there is the danger that the left and right side are disconnected. With the macrocosmic *E*, the human being can overcome this tendency of organic separation. Through this same force of the *E*, the growth of nerves is directed in such a way that the head and limbs are connected. 'This becoming *E* is thus summed up, this drawing oneself together into a point in the vertical, in the contour' of the spinal cord.

Stretching arises in the repetition of the *E* gesture. The predominant effect of the *E* first promotes the integration of the nerves, then this formative impulse turns away again – as in the description of the effect of the *O* – from the system of nerves and senses to the system of metabolism and the limbs; from the tendency to stretching in the spinal column arises the linear growth in the limbs. If this gesture of narrowing and stretching, through speech that is rich in *E*, remains effective even after the embryonic period, it can develop further only in the metabolism. Then there is a tendency to be a 'weakling,' and to anorexia.

In the examples of how *O* and *E* work during the organism's formative period, the development of head and nerves is referred to. This indication supports the classification in Chapter 3 of the vowels as they work on the upper human being. They do this as a cosmic impulse during the embryonic period and shape the nervous and sensory system above all. This occurs long before the vowels are heard or spoken. The vowels work later through one-sided speech (rich in *O* or *E*) with the same formative impulse, only in the wrong place: in the metabolism. They can work therapeutically when they are applied therapeutically in the right way as movement.

The idea that the cosmic vowels intervene formatively in the nervous system before birth may be extended hypothetically to include all the vowels. The nervous system is an instrument for the formative processes which work in out of the cosmos to build the body. The following considerations are suggestions for further investigation:

The cosmic *O* effects the 'centrifugal' growth of the nerve cells in the central nervous system. This force, which acts to extend in a direction from within outward, leads to a symmetrical rounding, to a sphere-forming process – the broadening and rounding of the head occurs. (See p. 91 of the Eurythmy Therapy Course).

The cosmic *E* effects the different crossings of the nerve pathways, the linking of the left and right halves of the body, and thereby the possibility for movements which cross. After the development of the crossed nervous system, the cosmic *E* leads to the stretching growth of the spinal column and the limbs.

The cosmic *I* keeps the organs of the median plane in their median symmetry, or combines potentially bilateral organs into a median (unified) one, for example the thymus gland.

The cosmic *U* enables the (laterally) symmetric development of organs, for example the parathyroid glands.

The cosmic *A* enables the development of bilateral organs out of a median predisposition, for example the lungs.

The cosmic vowel forces manifest in the formation of the organization. When the same vowel forces – for instance, through the frequent uttering of a vowel in a particular language – remain working for too long, vowel-specific one-sidednesses come about. These tendencies toward illness are stated for the *O* and the *E*; they probably apply for all the vowels.

The idea of polarity should be repeated: the cosmic consonant forces manifest in the building up force which leads to the growth of all organs. The cosmic vowel forces manifest in the shaping of the body. The organs are formed during the embryonic period through formation and growth, before they can function and serve the incarnating soul and self or I. The upper human being works in this shaping process from before birth, as the 'lower human being' works in growth. These forces should be employed in a healing capacity in eurythmy therapeutic activity.

The effect of eurythmy therapeutic vowel exercises is described in summary in the sixth lecture:

Those organs belonging to the rhythmic system are stimulated, the organs of respiration and the inner activity of digestion. These organs are strengthened; in them the appeal goes out to the forces of growth in the growing child, or ... to the plastic, sculptural [shaping] forces ... This will lead you into the physiology of doing vowels in eurythmy. (p. 76f).

The 'appeal' to the forces of growth, the impetus for building up, is always a function of the upper human being, because a new development is initiated through the 'appeal' (see Chapter 2). This impetus, descending from above, takes hold initially of the respiratory system, then of the inner digestive activity of the metabolism. (The circulatory system, which lies in between, has been skipped in this enumeration.) It is said later that, 'You can bring the human being organically to himself through doing vowels in eurythmy. You can awaken the forces that bring him to himself organically. For certain people this will be most necessary, among them sleepy-headed people.' (p. 85). The same formative and awakening upper forces can also be brought in by introducing sugar into the organism, as is stated just before the passage quoted.

In the seventh lecture, the effects of vowels working cosmically and through speech are correlated with processes of excretion. This appears to contradict the formative impulses as they have been described for all the vowels up to this point. In Chapter 13, an attempt will be made to work out what both indications have in common.

7.3   A suggested classification of eurythmy therapy indications for the vowels

In the following considerations, the therapeutic indications from the course will be drawn together and the attempt made to relate them to the whole human being. In doing so, the starting point will be similar to that adopted for the consonants, that the entirety of the vowels is related to the whole human being, and that the therapeutic indications described are only windows beyond each of which a corresponding world is to be found.

7.3.1   The I and U exercises

In the Eurythmy Therapy Course, the enumeration of the therapeutic effects of the vowels begins with the duality of *I* and *U*. The *I* should be practised with all those 'who cannot walk properly,' who walk clumsily. If someone were unable to walk with an energetic stride, their blood circulation would suffer as well. The following was mentioned as an additional, more psychical symptom in adults: The human being 'is somehow inhibited in expressing themselves properly, as a person. They might be a dreamer in a certain sense' (p. 16).

The *U*, on the other hand, is indicated for all people 'who cannot stand,' whose feet are weak and who tire easily when standing.

One can take as one's reference point the concrete, everyday processes of walking and standing. It becomes apparent that both conditions of movement continually and necessarily have to alternate. One walks for a bit, stops for one reason or other and remains standing; then one goes on again. 'Being able to walk' and 'being able to stand still' have their own rhythm and their own physiological limits for different people: everyone eventually has to cease active movement and return to a position of rest or even to recline. After a period of rest one needs to move again and walk. Usually the two states alternate in such a way that people can fulfil their intentions through either standing or walking. It becomes pathological when the flow of movement is disrupted by their slowing down or speeding up involuntarily. It is just as pathological if the rests or pauses which ought to punctuate the flow of movement occur involuntarily or cannot be maintained. Every course of movement is composed of a balance of flow of movement and periods of rest. Human movement is only conceivable as an alternation between active phases and longer or shorter pauses.

The unit of movement 'walking/standing' is probably again only an example, since all other movement processes are subject to the same principle. A painful limitation of movement in the shoulder joint would be a further example of 'not being able to move'; pathological blinking of the eyes, of 'not being able to remain still.' In the two examples neither the flow of movement nor the regular, necessary rest is sustainable. The human being cannot move enough ('not being able to walk') or they cannot maintain the necessary rests ('not being able to stand').

'Not being able to walk' can of course also be broken down into further polarities: a person is unable to walk because an excess of uncontrolled movement impulses impede the flow of movement, for example petit mal fits. Or they are unable to walk, because they are unable really to begin the movement, for example in Parkinson's disease. Conversely 'not being able to stand' can have different origins: on the one hand there might be an excessive restlessness of movement, which does not permit of standing; or someone might be unable to stand because fatigue or weakness inhibit an upright stance.

It is reasonable to proceed on the basis that every pathological variation of normal movement can be therapeutically influenced through the two vowels *I* and *U*. The *I* facilitates the physiological preconditions for movement processes; the *U* enables interruptions, pauses and rests. This assumption is supported by the way in which vowels are used therapeutically in the Curative Education Course: the 'weak-minded' child should bring their system of metabolism and limbs 'into movement' through the *I* (ee) in the sequence *R – L – S – I*; the 'manic,' hyperactive child has a *U* at the end of their sequence, in order to come to quiet.[9] In the eleventh lecture, the *U* should be employed 'in order to bring the astral body into strong, living activity, but in such a way that it is under control. And that's why the *U* is there.' The *U* is intended here to set a limit to the strong, living activity which leads to the movements.[10]

Kirchner-Bockholt mentions an exercise for scoliosis. The *I* should be done in a particular form in combination with *L*. The *L* is supposed to loosen what has become hardened; the *I* should be done with the arms and while hopping, in order to 'form [the flow of movement] in the right way.' One can also look in a similar way at the *I* in the sequence *G* – *K* – *A* – *I* for a child with a stutter, bedwetting and 'shaking of the head' (at night?). The flow of movement in the day should be achieved in speech. The *I* together with *L* – *M* should also be helpful for agoraphobia; walking is facilitated. Both vowels are recommended in the combination *L* – *I* – *M* – *A*, *R* – *U* for a patient with difficulty sleeping through the night and constipation, and who has cold feet and who fatigues quickly. It is understandable that the relation between moving and stopping, walking and standing should be influenced therapeutically here. All these examples support the suggestion of using these two sounds for the regulation of all movements and their necessary periods of rest.

The complex pattern of movement in being able to walk, stand or swim are described in the second lecture of the parallel medical cycle.[11] These complex movements are used as examples of how the I organization individualizes the system of metabolism and the limbs.

7.3.2   The O and E exercises

In the third eurythmy therapy lecture, a second duality is named: the *O* should always be applied when 'a child or adult is unnaturally fat.' The *E* stands at the opposite pole and should be applied for 'thinlings, that is to say for weak people.' In this description, the cause of the thinness does not seem to be crucial. It could be an organic illness or a psychic disorder. The *E* may well be done in different directions – forward or backward – but it remains *E*. (It may be assumed that the same differentiation is also valid for the *O*: *O* forward with more organic causes, backward when psychical problems predominate. This differentiation has proved valuable in practice.)

Again one can ask about the greater wholeness, into which these examples may be organized. Both indications for *O* and *E* have in common that a specific human process of building up substance has fallen into disarray: either too much or too little fat substance is formed.

Both disorders point to the formation of the human organism which is connected to lipometabolism. The normally formed human being has a healthy portion of fatty padding, which is as necessary for aesthetic appearance as it is for inner wellbeing.

> Fat is the substance in the organism which, when taken in from without, turns out to be the least foreign. This characteristic is only possible through its carrying over into the human organism the least possible of the qualities of a foreign organism, of its etheric forces, and so on.[12]

Fat is only slightly foreign and is easily stored. In short-term physical work it is not even metabolized. If a sufficiently intense, sustained
muscular effort is engaged, fat is enlisted as an energy source and warmth
is released. The fatty padding of the organism gives the potential for sustained efforts; it does not serve the needs of the normal metabolism of the
organism at rest. An overweight person is usually unfit; their high proportion of potential energy, trapped in their fat, contrasts with their limited
expenditure of effort. A slim person needs to take on nourishment at an
early stage in any strenuous effort, or they will start burning their own
bodily protein. Body fat only has a small part in everyday metabolism –
as everyone who would like to lose weight knows. A normal proportion
of fat is not an encumbrance and is available to the organism for extreme
efforts. Fat facilitates future efforts.

At this point, the question again arises as to whether the O and E are
only connected with this special kind of substance building and use, or
whether the building of fat is also just an example of a general rule. In
the narrow indication, the O is applied for overweight people. A possible generalization would be: substance-building in different areas of
the organism can be limited with the eurythmy therapy O. Could, for
instance, the amount of milk-secretion in a case of galactorrhoea be
reduced? Could an increased production of mucus in the intestine, or
a pathological production of sweat be regulated through the O? The O
could help in all illnesses where substances needed for special functions
are overproduced.

The polar process would then hold good for the E. In the narrow
indication, it should be applied for 'thinlings,' who cannot form enough
substance. The extension would be: it may be applied when the building of secretions, or of substances for specialized functions, either does
not begin or is not sufficiently strong. The E may be indicated when the
organism lacks the impetus to make secretions, and other substances
needed for specialized functions, in sufficient quantity.

E is frequently used to cut short a seizure.[13] In epilepsy, the balance
of building up and breaking down processes is disturbed: on the one
hand, certain nerve cells remain in a depolarized, excited state for too
long; on the other, the blood flow to the head and the supply of glucose
increases sharply during a grand mal fit. The interplay of stimulating
(exciting) and depressing (inhibiting) impulses, determined by messenger substances, is disturbed. The E engages therapeutically with this
interplay.

7.3.3   The A exercise

Before we examine the vowel A, a brief review may be helpful. In Steiner's indications for the consonants, the palate sounds G and H represent the force and potential of movement. If the vowels I and U are added, they point to the polarity between the flow of movement and its pausing or resting.

The teeth sounds D, S and Sh affect the metabolic processes of secretion and the building of substance used to activate different processes. The vowels O and E are also related to substances with a specialized function. They are used in cases of an excess or lack of fat formation as well as of other secretory processes.

The lip sounds B and F are used when the transformation of substances in the intestine is to be stimulated. With the consonants, the processes are followed from the outer, peristaltic movement in the intestine, through the necessary secretory processes of nourishment, to the point that substances cross the mucous membrane and enter the blood. Substances begin to be individualized.

The characteristic of the A can now be seen in connection with the following. In the metamorphosis of substances in the organism, they should first be enlivened from a mineral, fluid condition; then further enhanced to one which can carry soul elements; finally attaining a quality open to the self, the I. If this flow is interrupted, substances remain on a lower level, just etheric or just astral and animal-like; as substances which have been left behind their effect is pathogenic. The eurythmy therapy A helps in carrying the transformation of substance through all the levels of quality and into the openness for the I. In that respect it 'counteracts the animal nature.' The A helps the building of substance to reach the highest, human stage. The O and E are necessary to build or activate substances for a specialized function. The A helps the organism to individualize the substances inside the body.

7.3.4   The Au and Ei exercises

In speaking the Ei (as in 'eye') the formation in the mouth moves from A via E to the I, ranging up the left side of the vowel formations in Figure 4b. In the same way, the articulation of the Au glides from the A via the O to the U, combining the vowels spoken with a rounded tongue. These combining gestures of A–E–I or A–O–U support the idea that the therapeutic indications of Ei and Au are more central than the single vowels.

No-one asked a question about the therapeutic effect of either sound, although they were probably used, so there is no suggestion given by

Rudolf Steiner. The therapeutic indication can only be discovered by other means. The sequence of the previous investigation into the consonants, has also held good for the vowels up to now:

1. *Movement* becomes ordered with the consonants *K, G* and *H*, and with the vowels *I* and *U*.
2. *Secretion* and the forming of substances that carry a specialized function is ordered with the consonants *T, D, S* and *Sh*, and with the vowels *O* and *E*.
3. *Forming individualized substance* and the corresponding elimination are ordered with the consonants *P, B* and *F*, and with the vowel *A*.
4. The last step is taken with the consonants of the middle group *M/N, L* and *R*: the newly formed individualized substances are guided into and specialized for *the different organs*, where they serve building up processes according to their particular needs. The consonants create the forces for this building up. This consonantal part must everywhere be balanced through the formative processes which are enabled through the vowels. The functions of *Au* and *Ei* are the ordering of and setting of limits to the forces of growth.

We may assume that *Au* and *Ei* – like the other vowels – also have a formative effect during the embryonic period. The creative form impulses probably also have the integrating effect on a higher level, which stands out when they are spoken. The creative form impulses of the *Au* and *Ei* manifest in the whole form of the human being and of the individual organs.

This formation of the human being is described from two aspects in the lectures *Cosmosophy* (Vol. 2).[14] In one description the form impulses work directly and lead to the shaping elements of the upper human being, most clearly revealed in the rounding of the head. In the other, polar description, the limbs are formed through forces originating as metamorphosed cosmic forces that work through the earth.

The relation of the vowels to the planets has not so far been mentioned, so as to keep the investigation close to the Eurythmy Therapy Course. In the search for connections and contexts for the *Au* and *Ei*, this link may now be added to the considerations: *Au* is connected to the sun; *Ei* with the moon.

The forces related to the upper human being work out of the cosmos, the realm of the zodiac, via the moon, and are related to the *Ei*. This direct connection of the moon with the formative forces of the zodiac, described in the above lectures, is also to be found in the gesture for moon in eurythmy: it is at rest in itself like all the zodiac movements.

The seed-preserving forces which act formatively in the human being out of the earth are more strongly related to the sun and the *Au*.

As a eurythmy therapy exercise, the *Ei* has frequently proved valuable in cases of chronic pain. This is particularly the case for pain in the spinal column and for cancer patients with bone metastases. Care must be taken that, in the gliding movement of the *Ei*, the emphasis (character) remains in the peripheral parts and that the crossing itself is done with a limited tone in the muscles and remains unemphasized (movement). The conceptual integration of the *Ei* and experiences with patients reinforce each other: the inclusion of *Ei* in the cancer sequence is absolutely necessary (Chapter 14.1).

The *Au* is hardly used in eurythmy therapy.

7.4 Summary

The *I* facilitates the process of intentional movement.

The *U* enables the interruptions, pauses and rests which are a physiological part of movement.

The process of building substances used for specialized processes is limited through the *O*.

The *E* is indicated when the organism lacks the impetus to build sufficient secretions and other substances for specialized functions.

The *A* helps the building of substances to reach the highest, human stage, so that they can serve the self, or I.

The *Au* and *Ei* mediate, from the cosmos (*Ei*) and from the earth (*Au*), creative form-impulses which are necessary for the whole form (gestalt) of the human being and for the shaping of every individual organ.

8. Vowels and the Upper Human Being, Consonants and the Lower Human Being

In Chapter 2, we looked at the laws of the ether body. All living processes unfold in the tension between the upper and lower human being. The tendency to limit, to form and to break down proceed from the upper human being. The lower human being, by contrast, initiates all the processes of swelling and growth. A description from the Curative Education Course was summarized in Chapters 2 and 3. Vocalic eurythmy therapy stimulates the upper human being, while the opposite processes are activated by the consonant movements which reinforce the lower pole. We shall now look at what the consonant and vowel series have in common and what differentiates them.

8.1 Sounds influencing movements

The following descriptions have been made so far. First, the palate sounds *K, G* and *H* work on the movement of the gastrointestinal tract. Secondly, the *I* sound strengthens the capacity to carry out a flow of movement. The *U* mediates the capacity to maintain the pauses and rests which are part of movement.

Both these statements describe how the process of movement can be influenced. At the same time the duality of forces determining every function is highlighted.

On one hand a potential of energy has to be built up within the muscles, to allow movement, and the muscles must be maintained and built up anew after any exercise. This energy aspect can be allocated to the lower human being. The forces of movement in the whole organism are supported through the palate sounds *G* and *H*.

On the other hand, every movement needs to be shaped. This structure of a movement has a start, a flow and an end. The movement needs to be organized to result in a meaningful outcome. The peristalsis of the intestine, in addition to the force that comes from the lower human being, needs the organ-specific rhythm of contraction and relaxation. This rhythmic, shaping part of the movement corresponds to the activity of the upper human being. The timing and the ordering of the movement is mediated through the two vowels *I* and *U*. The *I* shapes the entirety of the complex process of movement, and can influence the particular muscular strength during a flow of movement. The *U*, by contrast, works on the ordering of the recovery phases and of the dilatation of all muscles during the pauses (Figure 6).

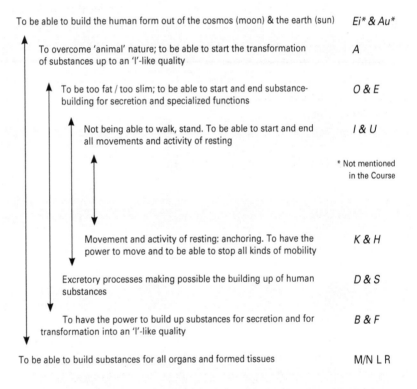

Vowels activate the forces of the upper human being

To be able to build the human form out of the cosmos (moon) & the earth (sun)   *Ei* & Au**

To overcome 'animal' nature; to be able to start the transformation   *A*
of substances up to an 'I'-like quality

To be too fat / too slim; to be able to start and end substance-   *O & E*
building for secretion and specialized functions

Not being able to walk, stand. To be able to start and end   *I & U*
all movements and activity of resting

* Not mentioned
in the Course

Movement and activity of resting: anchoring. To have the   *K & H*
power to move and to be able to stop all kinds of mobility

Excretory processes making possible the building up of human   *D & S*
substances

To have the power to build up substances for secretion and for   *B & F*
transformation into an 'I'-like quality

To be able to build substances for all organs and formed tissues   M/N L R

Consonants activate the forces of the lower human being

Figure 6. The working of vowels and consonants in physiological processes.

The effects of vowels and consonants

Vowels
forming, giving
impulses, ordering
and organizing out
of the upper human
being

Blown sounds
building up in the region
of the nerves and senses

Impact sounds
building up in the region
of the metabolism

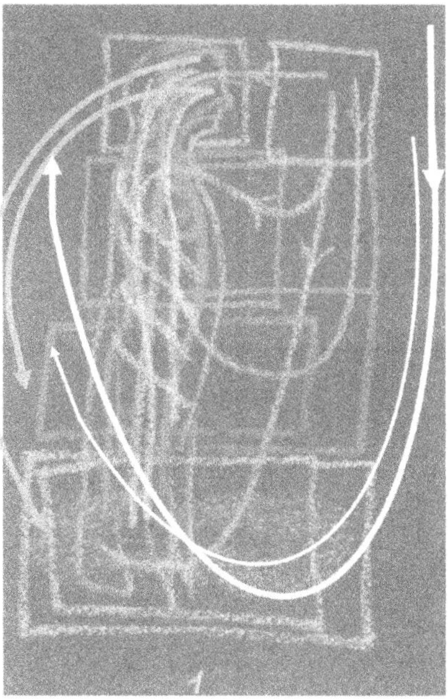

Figure 7. The workings of vowels and consonants in relation to the visible and the invisible human being

8.2 Sounds acting on the formation of substances with a specialized function

The following have so far been described. First, the teeth sounds *T, D* and *S, Sh* work on the preparation of secretions in the digestive tract so that the foreign nature of nourishment can be overcome. Secondly, the *O* is always indicated as a therapy when an excess of particular secretions, of fat or other substances is formed. The polar vowel, *E*, is helpful when substance formation or secretions are too weak.

These two statements describe a duality which can also be observed with every function of specialized substances. Both sides of secretion processes can be looked at. A very complicated process has to take place inside the glands or other tissues to build up the secretion. This building up process is ruled by the lower human being and can be harmonized through the consonantal teeth sounds.

On the other hand, a secretion can only start an appropriate function if it is secreted at the right time, if the fat can be used at the right time. This impulse to secrete and make available at the right time, in the right place and in the right quantity, is subject to the formative force of the 'upper human being.' The *O* leads therapeutically to a delimiting, the *E* to the beginning or strengthening of this forming process. The same relationship is shown in Figure 7, so that the therapeutic aims are identifiable, but now with the concepts from the lecture 'The Invisible Human Being in Us' (See also Chapter 16).

8.3   Sounds of transformation and individualization of substances

The following has been described up till now. First, the lip sounds *B* and *F* work on the force that enables foreign, mineral substances to be enlivened, and then in the realm of the kidneys to become carriers of soul, and finally to be refined in the liver to a quality that can carry the self, the I. Secondly, the *A* helps substance formation to attain the highest, human stage.

This duality has another aspect. The force in the organism through which the food that was initially foreign is raised and refined to a level that can serve the self, the I, is subject to the ordering of the lower human being. The lip sounds *B* and *F* mediate the driving forces which allow the higher development to human substance.

By contrast, the vowel *A* works from the level of the upper human being. It enhances the function allowing the organism to further refine only those substances that have been sufficiently transformed and are suitable for further development, thus preventing further development before the prior stage is complete. Here the shaping side of the process may be observed. The *A* structures the process of transformation; the lip sounds give the forceful impulse for this spiritualization of substance.

8.4   Sounds for organ-specific substance creation, the diphthongs *Au* and *Ei*

All the middle sounds, the *L* and *R* and the transition from these to the impact sounds *M* and *N*, activate the central processes of the ether body. They enable the building up of all the individual organs with the substances which have previously attained the capacity for carrying the self, the I, through the working together of the lip sounds and the *A*. In this way building up of bone and muscle, forming of nerves, and healing of wounds are achieved: the right substances have to be available at the right time in the right place. On the one hand the right substances have to be prepared, so that the appropriate building up processes can take place. This process belongs to the lower human being. The substances in the building up stream must be prepared properly, in order to be available for the specific building up in each organ. This building up process is supported through the middle sounds.

In a polar way, the *Au* and *Ei* mediate the impulses of form from the cosmos (*Ei*) and from the earth (*Au*) which are necessary for the whole form of the human being and for the structure of each individual organ, The upper human being again has to order and structure this building up process. The physiological processes involved in healing a wound must always take place in the right sequence. It is suggested that one draw on the activity of these two diphthongs for this central task of ordering and organizing – even though neither of them is mentioned in the course.

The organs have to be built during the embryonic phase long before they are able to start their function. Later on the organs can function and have to be remodelled or renewed regularly. The building up function is related to the teeth sounds and to *O* and *E*. The building up and shaping of the organs and their renewing every night is driven by the middle consonants *M/N, L* and *R* and the diphthongs *Au* and *Ei.*

9. The Soul Exercises

After the basic therapeutic laws of the vowel and consonant exercises had been developed, the soul exercises were introduced in Lecture 5 of the Eurythmy Therapy Course. Only after that were vowels and consonants joined in a therapeutic 'word' (Lecture 6).

The soul exercises were introduced as follows: 'Today we will turn to some of the eurythmical exercises more related to the activity proceeding from the soul' (p. 58). Doing this presupposes knowledge of how the movements of vowels and consonants are initially related to the working of the etheric. These exercises have in common that basic soul responses are to be activated through the eurythmy therapy movements. Up to now, the etheric processes have been evoked directly by consonant and vowel exercises. New soul experiences may have arisen in the patient indirectly. Steiner emphasizes this: 'Here we have a strong influence which proceeds from the human etheric acting on the astral' (p. 60). The new soul experiences, intended to be brought about through movements, strengthen the astral body first and work through the upper human being. In this, the soul exercises demonstrate their affinity with the vowel exercises. With these soul exercises, it is not necessary to evoke the awareness of resounding at the end, as in the vowel and consonant movements. Instead, polar reactions are evoked in the soul during each exercise and the soul's capacity to oscillate is extended. The movements of these exercises are described in detail by Glas.

9.1 Exercises with polar feelings

9.1.1 Forming judgments through thinking: affirming – negating

The first activity of the soul to be described is 'judgment'; the courage for decision has to be gained by this eurythmic exercise. Judgments are constantly arising in every human being. If one notices a traffic sign illogically placed, a typographical error, or if someone does not behave as expected, a judgmental response always arises in the soul: 'that's wrong, out of character, incomprehensible.' The human being becomes aware of a particular situation, of an error or discovery. The soul makes a judgment after a very brief reflection and comes to an inner negation or affirmation. This simple form of a judgment arising out of perception should be brought into a to-and-fro movement in the patient's soul through the eurythmy therapeutic movements. Patients often do not dare to rely on these spontaneous decisions. Courage is hereby aroused consciously to allow such judgments in the soul.

Soul experiences of this kind, which contain these polar elements, are not just to be taken up in the soul, but should be borne into the world visibly through movements. 'The movement ... works very strongly on the respiratory system by way of a detour through the etheric body' (p. 58). The life processes are therapeutically influenced out of the new soul activity *if shortness of breath is a symptom for a deeper pathological condition.* The way in which this effect comes about is described at length. Normally judgments spontaneously set off moods in the soul. For this one needs hardly any inner effort, that is hardly any I-activity. In any case, people's inner courage is not usually sufficient even to admit to these half-conscious, spontaneous judgments. The barely noticed fleeting thought contained in the judgment is guided into the limbs through the conscious movement's will effort. The limbs hereby become delicately subtly aware of the will element within the activity of judgment while the cause, the content of the judgment, withdraws from consciousness. This displacement of awareness from the head to the limbs, forms the ether body anew; an improvement in the breathing arises if the movements are done rapidly enough.

9.1.2 Agreement through the will: sympathy – antipathy

The second soul exercise is called 'agreement through the will.' Affirmation or negation arise here through the human soul spontaneously, as sympathy or antipathy, rather than as judgments bound up with thought. The dreamlike, nearly unconscious lethargy of the will cannot rouse itself to either sympathetic or antipathetic expression, is awakened through these movements. This lethargy of the will is overcome through the exercises with the limbs. 'The *I* is more strongly active in relation to the body than it usually is' (p. 60). This exercise in eurythmy therapy works indirectly on the circulatory system.

Through these movements, awareness of one's own feelings in the soul should become conscious and be strengthened. The movements work back in a second step on the living functions in an ordering and organizing way.

The starting point in both the previously described exercises is taken from polar soul gestures. No sounds are included yet. Activities of the soul, made conscious through the eurythmy therapy movements, unfold in the face of the polar gestures. The aim of these exercises is to encourage the soul to dare to decide 'yes–no' or 'I want – I reject.' The respiratory and circulatory system is stimulated indirectly through the upper organization.

The exercises for forming judgment and expressing the will may be combined if they are not sufficiently effective. Proportions of 2:3 or 3:2 are suggested for this. Both exercises have a wakening effect on the patient's soul life.

9.2   Feeling exercises and vowel exercises

9.2.1   Love–E

The next two exercises bring together vowel exercises and soul gestures. The love–E exercise will be considered first. In Section 7.1 the soul gesture which is experienced with the E was described as antipathy forces that impose limits and that enable an experience of the self. Steiner refers to the soul gesture in this way: 'E reveals a kind of holding onto oneself in the face of resistance.'[1] In these eurythmy therapy exercises the living forces which lead to movement are again evoked. Strong feelings – on the one hand of loving, through the love gesture; on the other of rejecting or setting limits through the E movement – are evoked in the soul. One is created out of an imagination, the other through doing a vowel exercise. Opposite soul forces are again brought to consciousness through the movements. A secondary effect 'really works on the circulatory system in a beneficial manner. One cannot say that it accelerates or retards the circulation, it affects it in a beneficial, warming way.' (p. 60). Living movements allow feelings to become clearer so that they can work back onto the processes in the sphere of life.

9.2.2   Hope–U

The following exercise takes its start once more from movements born out of a feeling and out of a vowel experience. In the first part of the exercise, the feeling of hope in the soul is evoked and strengthened through the movement. Then the vowel movement creates the U experience. Bort describes this: 'Fear and cold resound in the U, one's whole being draws together and becomes, as it were, hard and cold; deadly fear pervades.' Once more a gesture of opening is contrasted with the experience of drawing together in the *U*. The fear of an unknown future meets with hope, which can brighten the oppressive cares. In the previous example (love–*E*) it was emphasized that the effects of these soul movements transform the etheric and work into the astral. In this example, attention is drawn to the subsequent working back from the soul into the life sphere. 'The astral will act very strongly upon the etheric nature' (p. 61), and a beneficent, warming effect thereby engendered. The hope–*U* exercise is frequently employed in cases where there is a wish for children and where there is an intense longing for health.

In both exercises, balance of soul, which the patient probably wishes to strengthen in themselves, is practised through contrast: love and hope as feelings are initially intensified through the movements then contrasted with the polar soul gesture. The gesture of *love* with the delimiting *E*; the movement for *hope* with the fear-evoking *U*. The effect of both exercises is similar: from the gestures of a soul feeling and a vowel, a tension is created which activates the soul life and has a secondary effect on the ether body. The rhythmical system is strengthened: the love–*E* exercise works to harmonize the circulation; the hope–*U* exercise more on the rhythm of breathing. Within the rhythmical system, there is always an oscillation between action and reaction.

9.3 Laughter – *H–A*, Veneration – *A–H*

Soul gestures and eurythmy therapy sound-gestures are combined in a third way: in the next group of exercises, soul gestures are no longer expressed through movement; feelings are awakened in the soul and consciously ordered through eurythmy movements alone. In this way, a physiological healing effect unfolds. The right mood should arise in the soul through appropriate eurythmy therapy exercises only. If the sound sequence *H–A* is practiced in the right way, the mood changes towards laughter and lightness. The situation is different for the opposite sound sequence: when *A–H* is practiced rightly, the mood of veneration in the soul is strengthened.

The awakening condition of tension, which is evoked initially through the polar soul gestures (yes–no, sympathy–antipathy) and which is then metamorphosed through the polar tendencies of movements for feelings and of the vowels (love–*E*, hope–*U*), is further intensified. The effective field of forces in these exercises arises out of the polarity between consonant and vowel; they are combined into a little 'word.'

All soul exercises have in common that they work on the middle system of the human being: sometimes more in its lower part, the circulatory system; sometimes on the upper part, the respiratory system. The influence on the life processes occurs in each case through the awakening and strengthening of feelings in the soul, that is from the astral. Intensifying the soul activity creates the forces that make the ether body 'into a useful person'; the intervention in this group of exercises comes about invariably through resounding soul moods. These exercises are particularly suitable for clinical pictures characterized by a predominance of psychosomatic symptoms. For patients who are ill in this way, the interplay of their own soul reactions with their bodily symptoms is often not conscious. Soul experiences become more courageous and more conscious. This in turn leads to the rhythmical processes becoming more ordered again.

With this group of exercises, the replicating of the intoning or the imaging of the movement which have to be recalled in vowel or consonant exercises, are not necessary, but the concluding phase of sleep is.

10. Transforming Eurythmy into Eurythmy Therapy

10.1 The connection between moving and speaking or listening

In different places in the Eurythmy Therapy Course and the Speech Eurythmy Course, the beginnings of the development of speech are referred to, as a close relationship exists between speech and the system of movement: 'In truth, the whole of speech arises through movement of the human limbs which has been held back.'[1]

Steiner described how in the very early stages of humanity, speaking or listening to speech was still closely bound up with movements of the whole body; a corresponding movement of the limbs or the whole body was part of every spoken utterance. And the other way round: when a movement of the limbs was intended, this was expressed with sounds. Only a scanty remnant of this still lives in the gestures which today accompany speaking or listening. In the course of the development of humanity and of speech, the relationships of vowels and consonants to their corresponding human movements have changed. The vowels became more closely bound up with feelings in the soul. In speaking they were thereby 'taken quite far into the human being's inner world.' The corresponding movements of the limbs were reduced to movements in the larynx and the rest of the speech instrument, so that any visible expression was almost completely lost. Through the imbalance between speaking and moving that arose thereby, the situation comes about today that speaking a language rich in O leads to one-sidedness, of the soul and the body. The physiological result which develops unconsciously from speaking the O is obesity as described in Section 7.2. A language rich in E effects the opposite: 'A language that is rich in E will engender skinny people' (p. 38).

It is indicated here that speaking the vowels O and E is always bound up with the tendency to lead to one-sided or even pathological changes in the organism. We can assume that this tendency to one-sidedness also holds good for other vowels, even though this is not mentioned in the text. Speaking the *O* increases existing obesity, which is countered through the eurythmy therapy exercise. The same thought process would hold good for the other vowels: through speaking them, one-sidednesses and pathological tendencies arise which are in turn overcome through the intoning of, moving to and listening for the vowel in question. Speaking *U* causes 'not-being-able-to-stand'; speaking the *I*, the danger 'of not being able to walk properly.' Speaking the *A* causes one-sidedness making it more difficult to sustain transformation. Substances do not adequately lose the character of the world outside, so the inner quality is not sufficiently developed.

In therapeutic exercises, the patient first speaks aloud the vowel which increases the pathological tendency. Then, in the eurythmy therapy exercise, the limbs are engaged in the vowels; finally, the vowel should be listened for (Section 10.2.1).

The relation to the consonants, on the other hand, has developed in the opposite direction. Here, too, the original concordance between moving and speaking or listening has been lost. The speaking and hearing of consonants is today accompanied by movement only to a slight extent, and corresponding feelings no longer resonate in the soul. The movements of the consonants cannot be described as soul qualities, like those of the vowels. To characterize a consonant movement, images from nature have to be created within the soul, for example the *w*elling of *w*ater, the *b*uilding a *b*ower, and so on. The consonants have been externalized – so it was described – too far into the surrounding formations of nature; the relation to movement and to the human being's feelings has largely been lost. Later in Lecture 6 it is described that people who have to listen to much that is consonantal, develop peculiarities. Originally the human being used to move in sympathy while hearing the movement-images of the consonants. This need to express the gestures belonging to the consonants was lost at the same time as were the movements accompanying the speaking of vowels. The predominant hearing of consonants – without their accompanying gestures – leads to a will that is blocked, that cannot live itself out. 'Listening to consonants is inwardly exceptionally invigorating ... You may notice an intensification of self-assertion and self-will in people who are accustomed to living in the consonantal element. (pp. 78, 80). This inner strength can intensify further into aggression. This self-will manifests first more on a soul level, but later also bodily as a tendency to illness.

Unfortunately there is no differentiation at this point as to which forms this self-will can assume, depending on whether a language is rich in blown sounds or in impact sounds. It may be assumed that here too there is a spectrum of pathological tendencies that develop, specific to the different sounds.

Listening to individual consonants leads to one-sidednesses, both of soul and of body. The consonant exercises can heal particular pathological tendencies. Uttering individual vowels leads to one-sidednesses of soul and body. The vowel exercises can heal particular pathological tendencies.

In eurythmy therapy, tendencies that lead to illness should be taken hold of consciously and transformed through the right movement. The disjuncture which developed out of the vowels' being too strongly internalized and the consonants' being too strongly externalized needs to be overcome. The development of humanity led them out of paradise. On this path, the harmony of movement and speech was lost in two directions. Eurythmy therapy has the task of bridging this gap and combining movement and speech again in a new way.

10.2 The sequence of the eurythmy therapy exercises

10.2.1 The sequence of the vowel exercises

In the second and fourth lectures attention is drawn to how the vowel and consonant exercises are built up in fundamentally different ways. With the vowel exercises, the first step is that the patient should sound the vowel aloud and at length; they should intone it. After that the exercise is carried through as movement, 'when they [the patients] have done that, you should try to to call forth in them [the impression] that they hear the sound that they have just carried out, as if they heard it' (p. 55). At the end of the exercise, the vowel should be experienced echoing in the soul in sound and movement.

The vocalic exercise consists in the first instance of the three steps: First sounding, secondly moving, and thirdly inner echoing or listening afterward.

What changes may be looked for in the organism through each of the three steps? Through speaking or intoning the sound, the one-sidedness that causes illness is intensified; speaking the *O* increases obesity, and so on. The vowels as cosmic sounds originally worked in a shaping, formative way into embryonic development. In this time before birth, the human being cannot yet intone vowels. Later in life the one-sided speaking of vowels that has been reduced from a cosmic formative force to an isolated movement in the speech instrument, works on in the same way: the *O* 'broadens, rounds out.' Only, this tendency no longer works in the right place – the head – but now occurs in the metabolism and leads to obesity. All vowels work similarly.

Through intoning the vowel at the beginning of the exercise the pathological tendency is initially intensified.

Then the actual movement exercise is carried out with the limbs. This follows a clear sequence, particularly for the 'great vowel exercises.' The individual sound should be moved first with the arms – repeated several times – then it should be done with the arms swinging swiftly, and later with the legs. The arm exercise should be done before and after the leg movements. A certain state of fatigue should set in. The energy for the leg exercise should be about a third of that of the whole movement. Following the intensification of the one-sidedness in the initial intoning, now fatigue and a breaking down process (through burning energy) in the limbs is induced.

The next step is the inner echoing. A conscious inner perception of the sound intoned earlier should resound in the soul. This resonance is a mental image called up through memory. The exercise becomes effective only if there is a strong impression. Delicate breaking down processes in the nervous system take place whenever we act consciously, as in this mental effort.

The breaking down process is active in all three steps of the vowel exercise. It begins from the speech organism; then takes hold of the limbs in fatigue; and finishes with conscious concentration on a memory-image. The whole human being is influenced by this breaking down. The effect of a particular vowel exercise is imprinted in certain parts of the body. During the succeeding period of rest or sleep, our higher self, the I of night-time, will become aware of the imprints and can work on these parts therapeutically building up with the cosmic vowel forces. The healing, therapeutic impulse only sets in during the recovery phase. The importance of the period of rest after the eurythmy therapy exercise will be explained in more detail later.

So the complete vowel exercise consists of four steps. First the patient intones the sound – sounding; secondly moving the arms – legs – arms; thirdly inner echoing of the sound which one has intoned and moved; and fourthly, the the phase of rest.

10.2.2 The swiftness of the consonant exercises

The suggestions in the text of the Eurythmy Therapy Course as to whether the exercises should be done quickly or slowly appear at first glance to be unsystematic.

As far as concerns the impact sounds, *D* & *T* and *B* & *P* should be carried out for some minutes until fatigue sets in. Fatigue will only set in if the exercises are done sufficiently fast.

G & *K* alone have no analogous indication.

With the blown sounds, it is said for *H* and also for *Sh* that the exercise should be done slowly and with pauses. 'It is important for the *H* and the Sh movements that they be done slowly.'

Nothing is specified for the *F*.

In the middle sounds, *R* is clarified such that the exercise should be done for a few minutes and several times a day.

If these few indications are integrated into the organization that has been built up for the consonants, the missing details in the mosaic may be adduced.

— The impact sounds should always be done quickly and until fatigue sets in.
— The middle sounds should be done for minutes at a time and several times a day.
— The blown sounds should be carried out slowly and with pauses; but the accentuation at the beginning of the exercise – the character – must be with sufficient emphasis.

10.2.3 The sequence of the consonant exercises

A fundamental difference in the sequence of the consonant exercises compared to that of the vowel exercises is described in the second lecture.

In the case of consonants, it is particularly important to have not a feeling in the way one does with a vowel, a feeling of stretching, of bending, or of widening, and so on, but to imagine oneself simultaneously in the form that one carries out while doing the consonant, as though one were to observe oneself.

... when you have a child or a grown-up carry out something having to do with consonants, it is important that they, as it were, photograph themselves inwardly in their thought; then in this inward photographing of themselves lies that which is effective. The person must really see themselves inwardly in the position that they are carrying out; it has to be carried out in such a manner that the person makes an inner picture of what they do. (p. 26).

Just as, with the vowel movements, the inward listening afterwards stands at the end of the whole process, so with the consonant exercises, besides the outer movement, one's own inner activity should be experienced and observed. The patient must be led and methodically guided toward this. It is important that the movement exercises of the consonants are accompanied by a conscious observing. 'In this inward photographing of themselves lies that which is effective.'

The complete structure of the consonantal exercises is only hinted at in this lecture. The aim consists in internalizing the consonants through moving the arms and legs simultaneously, and in the simultaneous, image-like, inward experience of these movements. What steps need to be taken in building up the exercise so that the patient can find the way to this goal? To find an answer to this, the difference between vowels and consonants must again be mentioned. In the structure of the vowel exercise, the patient begins with the intoning. The vowel is sounded without any movement. The obese patient intones the *O*, the thin one the *E*, and so on, and in doing so intensifies the one-sidedness. Following that, the movement that has been 'forgotten,' but which is being inwardly sought as a counterbalance, is carried out with the limbs. Ultimately moving and intoning should be consciously experienced in unison once more. This commonality was natural in ancient times; in the current state of development it should not simply be repeated outwardly, just by simultaneously moving and intoning. Neither the therapist nor the patient should speak and move simultaneously. The harmony of intoning and moving should be generated consciously by force of will through listening afterward; they should be united anew. What was originally, in the beginnings of the development of speech, a spontaneous simultaneity should now be built up in conscious awareness as a new unity: the harmonizing of the spoken sound with the movement belonging to it and bearing the signature of the individual soul.

With the consonants, the relationship of the sound and its corresponding movement develops in a polar opposite way to the above. What is expressed in speech is not internalized here. The consonant, as an experience within the soul, has been almost completely forgotten. Admittedly it is visible in the movements of nature, but it is not seen as such. The forces of the consonants have scarcely any relationship to the soul's experience any more. The consonant has been 'too strongly externalized.' The consonants should be internalized again in the eurythmy therapy exercises. Here too an earlier stage of development should be attained on a new level: the unity of the heard consonant and the movement done should be experienced inwardly and thus engendered anew in consciousness. How are consonant exercises built up didactically?

It is to be assumed that, with the consonant exercises, one may also start from the one-sided state prevalent today. The vowel exercises began with the sounding of the vowel, thereby strengthening the tendency to illness. By the same token, the consonant exercise can begin by first bringing to the patient an image from nature. They should see and become familiar with movement processes in living nature. This activity of nature should again and again be recalled from memory and wondered at. It could be the loud impact of a drop of water in a cave of stalactites (*T*), or the enfolding gesture of a bud scale or a bird's nest (*B*). Lory Maier-Smits reports on how the sound *L* was introduced:

> With *L*, one should always try to become aware, everywhere in nature, of the capacity to unfold freely ... This may be provided most clearly by the plant world. Gripping and the gathering of forces in the region of the roots; carrying up sap through the stem; the unfolding of leaves; the lighting-up of the blossoms; and at last sinking back into the earth in withering. You need to be able to bring to life the course of a whole year in this movement.[2]

A genuine process in nature, not a technical one, is built up out of the patient's wealth of experience. To begin with, the consonant is neither spoken nor heard. The therapist helps in filling out the picture; they correct the movements out of their knowledge of nature's processes and of the movement of the sound. The nature image is joyfully formed and shaped by the patient. Only much later, when the movement of the arms and hands really imitates the natural event, does the nature image withdraw into the background, and the therapist speaks the sound or also forms it themselves. Otherwise, if the patient hears the sound too soon, there is a danger that they will speak it as well, inwardly. When speaking silently, inwardly, the speech instrument is moved delicately in sympathy. Simultaneous movement of speech instrument and limbs weakens the eurythmy therapeutic effect (Section 11.2). The patients experience themselves in the consonantal movement and can also observe this experience inwardly.

The one-sidedness, brought on by the externalization of the consonants, is once more intensified. The movement arises from the nature image. Arms and legs form the consonant until fatigue sets in. At the same time an inner experience arises in the patient that the nature of the consonant may be beheld within them, it becomes visible to the imagination. This is called 'photographing' in the Course.

The didactic structure of the consonant exercises consists initially of three steps.

1. The patient imagines an image from nature and moves it; they thereby get to know the movements in nature of the consonants. The sound itself accompanies this process unconsciously; it is not yet audible. The therapist does not speak it yet.

2. The eurythmy therapist speaks the sound; the patient hears it outwardly and inwardly and moves it with the arms and legs simultaneously. They begin to experience themselves in the process of the consonantal movement.

3. The patient shapes the movements of their limbs and allows the doing and the heard sound to become conscious – simultaneously with the outer movements.

The *consonants* have become too externalized in the evolution of the human being; no soul experience resonates when one hears them; the images in nature have been lost. The correct movement of the sound draws the movements in nature toward the human being once more. Through this, the consonants are united again with the essential nature of the human being through the will. The sound is then brought into consciousness through willed beholding and through hearing.

The *vowels* have become too internalized. Through movement, they are brought into the limbs and subsequently into consciousness through the listening afterward. Through this, the feelings connected with the vowels are externalized. Movement and spoken sound combined can become effective again. Herein lies the healing power of eurythmy therapy.

The heard consonants (with their tendency to make one-sided) are internalized again from nature into the human being, through the eurythmy therapeutic movements of the consonants. Through this they attain the power to heal.

The spoken vowels (with their tendency to make one-sided) are liberated again from the soul through the eurythmy therapeutic movements of the vowels and become outwardly visible. Through this they attain the power to heal.

In the case of the therapeutic 'word,' where vowel and consonant appear together, neither the consonantal nor the vocalic form of internalization may be practised in their pure form. It is a question as to how the internalization of the consonants and the externalization of the vowels may be brought to a new harmony.

10.3 The four steps of transformation from eurythmy to eurythmy therapy

In this section the different conditions will be examined which must be observed when the movements which have been learned for artistic eurythmy are to be transformed for therapy. To start with general differences will be described before tackling the central task: how are the elements of eurythmy (movement, feeling and character, described in Chapter 4) to be transformed? These three basic elements are also valid for eurythmy therapy. They can in each case be taken hold of anew and transformed, in order that the moved sounds may unfold their therapeutic power.

10.3.1 Arms and legs

In the first lecture of the Eurythmy Therapy Course, the *I–A–O* exercise is introduced. In the following lecture a difference between eurythmy and eurythmy therapy is mentioned: the eurythmy therapeutic exercises should be done with arms and legs. 'In health-promoting eurythmy it would be good to have the movements – which are carried out with the arms only in artistic eurythmy – carried out with the legs as well where possible' (p. 22f). The whole body should be moved in the one sound. The exercises with the legs can be done simultaneously with those for the arms, or rhythmically alternating. They can be made as movements of the feet or of the whole legs. The individual sound movements can initially be prepared while sitting or while standing on one leg, so that the free leg can practice and learn the sound. The greatest intensification is achieved by jumping or by hopping: the sound is formed with the legs during the jump itself. This is the most difficult: in the brief moment free of gravity the sound movement should be accomplished with the legs.

The characteristic movements of the sound carried out with arms and legs also hold good for the *L* hopping. In the description of the exercise it may indeed say: 'Now an *L*; here again together with the effort to place the legs in the knock-kneed position and hop forward' (p. 50). The *L* with the legs begins with the starting position which is generally described as knock-kneed. With this starting position, the form-in-movement of the *L* can described by the legs while hopping.

Another kind of leg movement can be made if the sound is moved as a form in space. The form of the vowel can be carried out spatially by the patient stepping, alone or with others. This possibility of representing the sound by stepping does not arise with the consonants. Why do the inwardly experienced vowels have an outer form in space, while the 'externalized' consonants do not? Why are there for all the vowels the corresponding movement forms which are stepped, and nothing corresponding for the consonants?

The forming of the sound movements with the legs frequently appears grotesque and hardly elegant. Beauty is not the important thing. What matters is that the sound movements imprint themselves onto and transform the person's whole body, the arms above as much as the legs below.

When building up the exercise, it may be taken as a matter of course that the leg movements of the consonants or vowels be practised initially independently of the arm movements. The eurythmy therapeutic effect probably increases gradually; the more freely and the better the sound movements of the legs and the arms occur simultaneously, the more intense the therapeutic effect. One cannot, of course, expect every patient to manage the intensification into the jump.

10.3.2 Rapid repetition

A second criterion which distinguishes eurythmy therapy from eurythmy has to do with the order of the movement. The same sound movement is to be done repeatedly, as many times as possible, rapidly in succession. One notices that muscular tension increases during the rapid activity and that the character is intensified. This is desirable. The repetition of the same thing, as well as the speed or acceleration during the repetition, lead quickly away from artistic eurythmy. In the rapid repetition, the individual sound is experienced less and less out of an artistic intention. Instead, the impulse to move arises increasingly out of a dream-like momentum of habit. The soul's awareness, its experience of itself, is subdued during the rapid movement. If the sound has inscribed itself a little into the habits of the body through the rapid movement, the consciousness must be even more awake afterward: in listening afterward to the vowel exercise and in the picture experience of the inner photographing.

10.3.3 Practising and fatigue

Through the rapid repetition of the sound at some length, a further difference to artistic eurythmy is effected: the individual exercises should be carried out until the onset of more or less intense fatigue. The details of the sound are already disappearing during the rapid repetition. In addition, the patient becomes tired and warm through the intense movements of the sounds. The following is said for the *O* exercise: 'But at the same time ... it is of special significance that you have the person practise only as long as they can without sweating heavily and becoming too warm' (p. 19). This reservation is understandable with patients who are overweight, as they more quickly reach the limits of what they can achieve. With other patients, the particular exercise – adapted for the individual patient – may well be continued until perspiration begins or they are unable to continue. Fatigue occurs physiologically through the breaking down of energy-rich substances in the muscle; at the same time heat is generated. The breaking down process in the muscles and the associated development of heat occur in a manner specific to the sound and shows the imprinting activity. This vowel-like or consonant-like breaking down creates the precondition for the following building up healing, occuring in the rest or sleep following the eurythmy therapy exercise.

10.3.4 Alertness during the exercise

A fourth step of transformation from eurythmy to eurythmy therapy is mentioned in the second lecture: ' it is very important that we develop a feeling for what flows in the movement ... that tells us whether what is happening in the respective limb is a stretching, a rounding, or some such. One must decidedly acquire a specific consciousness for this.' (p. 15). The movement, the posture or the muscle tone should be felt with the movement sense; they should be shaped consciously. It was even said for the *O* exercise that the patient should have a consciousness of their being fat. 'It is particularly important ... that the eurythmy-therapy exercise is strengthened by extending it into the consciousness ... The element of consciousness is not in the least to be underestimated in healing.' (p. 119). So consciousness is required in four places:

1. In the first stage of practising, the vowels should be consciously intoned, and the consonants imagined consciously as a nature image and then heard.

2. During the exercise movement and character should be felt and con-sciously experienced. The character applies on the one hand to the ending position for the vowels and impact sounds, on the other to the beginning of movement with the blown sounds. There the character appears visibly.

3. After the eurythmy exercise, memory images should be built up in the form of inwardly hearing the vowels and building up of a picture of the consonant ('photographing'), as the third step of the exercise.

4. The patient should not suppress their being ill, but recognize it and be an active collaborator in their recovery.

10.3.5 Summary

The transformation of eurythmy into eurythmy therapy should be practised in four different ways. The individual elements are to be applied
individually, according to the individual patient and according to the illness. They must be practised one after the other, but the aim is that all four
elements be applied vigorously:

1. The movements of the sounds should be made with the arms and legs.
   In this way, the whole body is penetrated by the sound gesture; the
   body is filled and imprinted with the power of the vowel or consonant. This is the spatial aspect.
2. The exercises should be drawn out over time through rapid repetition.
   The individual sounds do not appear just once; they are not just hinted
   at, as in forming the words in artistic eurythmy; rather they become
   habitual through repetition and weeks of practice. They are inscribed
   into the ether body.
3. The exercise should be continued until the onset of (greater or lesser)
   fatigue. The breaking down effect manifests in tiredness of the limbs
   or of the whole body. This breaking down should take hold of the
   patient's whole will-sphere, in the ensuing period of rest, the the
   building up parts of the human being can bring healing according to
   the particular sound. The building up forces are brought to the location where healing is needed.
4. At the end the exercise should be raised clearly into consciousness.
   Each individual step of the exercise puts its own challenge to the clear
   awareness of the doer. This part of the exercise will only succeed if
   the eurythmy therapist has herself experienced it with all its difficul-
   ties and can thus guide the patient to an individual experience. This
   conscious conclusion to the exercise succeeds only when the 'I' of the
   therapist and the patient are fully present.

10.4 Processes of the day and the night to be activated in the ether body

In the previous section we stated that in all the individual steps of the
eurythmy therapy exercises, pathological tendencies are initially intensified and breaking down processes aimed at.

First, during the intoning of the vowels and the building up of a consonant image and the corresponding listening, one-sidedness is intensified.
Every exercise takes its start from the current situation: the vowels and

consonants have been separated from their original, resonating movements; in this way their tendency to one-sidedness is taken up.

Secondly, in practising the movements with arms and legs to the point of fatigue, energy and bodily substance are broken down in ways specific to particular sounds. The limbs are imprinted with the sounds.

Thirdly, in all processes of consciousness, and particularly in the effort to create either a more pictorial or a more auditory mental image after the exercise, imprinting and breaking down processes are induced in the nervous system.

Through all these steps, the higher supersensible members of the human being are activated in such a way that they have an immediate breaking down effect. The vowel or consonant is taken up in the realm of hearing and speech; they are worked at with the limbs until fatigue ensues and until they become habit; finally the specific shape or form of the vowel or consonant is embedded in the nervous system as the content of a mental image. If the sound is practised purely and with facility, the breaking down in the limbs and nervous system is shaped in such a way that, for a higher awareness, the archetypal form of the sound becomes perceptible in this breaking down. In the period of rest which follows, the daytime I is released out of the body. It moves out into the cosmos and takes with it, into the world of the planets and zodiac, the experiences specific to that sound, which it has won as the daytime I.

The more clearly and regularly the breaking down processes have been imprinted through practice in their sound-specific way during the day, the better the night-time I can reach the archetypes. The building up in the body only occurs in the period of rest or at night during sleep, in such a way that both the shaping, formative forces and the burgeoning, renewing forces which have the capacity for germination can intervene in a healing way. The phase of rest after the exercise is an indispensable part of the exercise. The building up, night forces can only work during sleep in a healing way, after the exercise has caused the breaking down.

As few sense-impressions as possible should be taken in between practising the sounds and the succeeding phase of rest. The room for resting should be close by; noise should not disturb the time of rest.

10.5 Transformation of movement, feeling and character into eurythmy therapy

Just as the sculptor controls the surfaces, the reciter shapes the sounds and the musician the tones, in order to achieve their purpose, so too the eurythmist must achieve everything that can be attained, using movement, feeling and character. Nothing further may be considered. This is the realm of eurythmy's artistic media. Through these everything must be accomplished.[3]

These statements relate to artistic eurythmy. We pointed out earlier that the description of the elements of eurythmy did not happen until a year after the Eurythmy Therapy Course. So the question arises as to how far the three elements movement, feeling and character are described in that course. The description from Chapter 4 will now be taken further for eurythmy therapy.

Up till now, four criteria have been mentioned to establish the distinctive features of eurythmy therapy as opposed to artistic eurythmy. They apply for all eurythmy therapeutic vowel and consonan exercises.

1. The sound movements are extended spatially to arms and legs, to the whole body.
2. The exercises are expanded in time through repetition of the same movement in a rhythmical way.
3. The individual exercise is practised until fatigue sets in.
4. The individual exercise should finally be pictured again as a unity of (spoken or heard) sound and the experience of movement.

In training the eurythmic capacity to form a sound, the *movement* element is generally practised first, through imitation. Then *character* is experienced ever more distinctly. Perception of the forces of the periphery – suction and pressure from the surroundings – is finally taken into one's practice, in order to learn the experience of *feeling*. Practising the movements of the sounds, on the one hand, and the inner monitoring of all the elements of movement during practice, on the other, form the sensory, living foundation of eurythmic movement. Through the senses of touch, movement, balance and life, the movements are inwardly imprinted and gauged; in this way, they can be enhanced in a continual learning process and the approach to the sound can be expanded. The sensory (synaesthetic) symbioses, which belong to the sounds in their threefold colouring open up the approach to the sounds through imagination. This spiritual approach is enhanced through knowledge of the sound's connection with the cosmos, described in spiritual science. Moving eurythmically becomes a path of practice to find the creative beings who are a part of the logos, as Martin-Ingbert Heigl points out.

This connection lives in every eurythmy therapist through the basic eurythmy training. When they practise with a patient, the latter should not at first see the coloured wooden eurythmy figure. Otherwise there would be a risk that they might unconsciously copy it in their movements. This would prevent them from experiencing the processes in their own body when they practise. Nor, too, should the realm of symbiotic colour experiences be shared with them through explanations; this should rather be experienced directly by the patient in their imitative doing. Admittedly, this is only possible when the therapist's own perception of the elements movement, feeling and character lives strongly enough in their soul.

To make this clear, every eurythmist may ask the following questions: how far do I succeed in perceiving the weight and lightness in the movement of the sound *I*, so that orange lights up in my soul as a sensory symbiosis? Can I perceive the field of tension between suction and pressure (and other forces from the periphery) for the sound *I* in such a way that the red of the sound *I* is experienced in the soul synergistically? Can I grasp the tensing and relaxing of the muscles in movement in such a way that the blue of the character of the sound *I* is created in my soul as a sensory symbiosis?

10.5.1 Transformation of the movement element

The three elements of eurythmy (movement, feeling and character) were described in Chapter 4. Steiner characterizes as movement the part that appears visibly. This is directly perceptible; it is always recognizable even in film and in isolated experimental conditions. The spatial and chronological aspects of a human movement are viewed in the element of movement. In isolation, movement has only a minimum of muscle tension. During the movement, the working of gravity is experienced more or less strongly.

At the end of a eurythmy therapy exercise, fatigue or mild perspiration should set in. Both the fatigue and the perspiration induce a languorous heaviness in the limbs. At the same time, every new beginning of the exercises brings with it an experience of the lightness of the exercise already practised earlier. Through the more conscious experience of heaviness and lightness during the movement, eurythmy is enhanced to eurythmy therapy. The repetition of the exercise and the expansion of it to include both arms and legs also enhances this element.

When practising eurythmy therapy it is good if the fatigue is clearly experienced at the end of each therapy session. Compared to eurythmy, the element movement must be enhanced and intensified in eurythmy therapy.

10.5.2 Transformation of the feeling element

The element of feeling, the veil, describes the perception of the periphery during eurythmic movement. This element of movement is experienced as a sucking or barely perceptible tug, or as a gentle touching or pressing from outside. This suction or pressure changes when different nuances of feeling (that is the colours of the figure) should be experienced or formed.

There is a place in the Eurythmy Therapy Course that could refer to feeling, to the veil movement, with consonants. Taking *Ha* and *eF* as an example, the following is said: '*H*: here you have an energetic unfolding into the outer world; ... one wants to go out and live in the external world. *F*: you see the decided effort to avoid entering into the outer world too sharply, to remain in the inner experience' (p. 31). This statement relates to eurythmy practice: the space around should be experienced with a differentiated intensity and integrated into the movement. In an experimental approach, different experiences can be made depending as to whether the *eF*, or the *Fe* (*Phi*) as the Greek *F*, are practised eurythmically. The German *Ha* and the English *Aitch* need to be expressed differently, because the space around the eurythmist is integrated differently.* In both kinds of sound-movement, the experience of heaviness and lightness, that is the movement, and of tensing and relaxing, that is the character, remain largely similar in both kinds of sound-movement.

With the *Fe*, the eurythmic shaping and forming requires the doer to feel drawn right out into the periphery. 'I am right out in the periphery and feel my boundaries from without.' This description goes for all consonants that sound with the vowel after (*Ka, Te, De, Pe, Be, Ve* and the German *Ha*): the self of the eurythmist experiences itself in the element feeling or veil wafting in from the outside, from the periphery, halting at the boundaries determined by character.

With the *eF*, this force of the feeling element from the periphery is less strong. The experience here can be described as 'I expand my inner world into the surroundings.' With the aspect feeling, the I of the eurythmist experiences the periphery nearer to their own figure, going

---

* Whether the English *H* is expressed eurythmically like the German *H* or whether this 'unfolding into the outer world' with the feeling (veil) is different because of the different pronunciation of this sound is still open to debate.

out more from their own centre. The veil wafts less strongly from the far distance of the periphery than with the *Fe*, and more in the immediate surroundings. It touches the movement and character of the sound. This shaping of the feeling applies to *eM*, *eN*, *eL*, *eR*, *eF*, *eS* and the English *H* [*Aitch*].

The tension of suction and pressure from without must be consciously grasped by the eurythmist for this differentiation of the consonants with vowel before or after, in order to make this detail visible. This element is the most difficult to learn when training for eurythmy. The capacity to make this element visible in the different colours determines the power of expression of eurythmy as an art. In eurythmy therapy, the patients should direct their complete attention and will-to-practise to the exact movement and to the character. The veil remains unseen. Even the eurythmy therapist discovers through intensive therapeutic activity how much the element of feeling withdraws.

10.5.3 Transformation of the character element

The third element of eurythmy or eurythmy therapy is called character: 'You tauten your forehead ... you feel you are bringing energy into the muscles of the upper arm; or you consciously position your feet while pressing down on the floor ... That is the third element, "character".'[4]

The experience of one's own strength is brought into eurythmic activity and shaped there. Through this, one's own will is experienced as activity. At the beginning of the educational work eurythmists did not take sufficient notice of this will element.

In the Eurythmy Therapy Course in 1921, the necessity of emphasizing character in eurythmy therapy was only hinted at:

Bear in mind that the person concerned, the person who carries out these things in order to enter therapy, feels them. In *E* you feel that one arm covers the other ... In *O*, feel not only the closing of the circle, but the bending as well. You feel that you are forming a circle. (p. 20).

In the Stuttgart lecture it is stated more clearly in the description of the *O* exercise:

All these forms, if they are intended to bring results as eurythmy therapy, must be combined with a distinct perception of the muscular system involved ... It will not have a therapeutic effect, unless in the process of doing the exercise you feel the muscles throughout the arm. The slack swinging form has no effect; the sensation of the whole muscular system in its details, however, will bring the respective therapeutic-eurythmical result. (p. 119).

The character of a eurythmy therapy movement is intensified when the muscles are felt in all their details – more strongly than in eurythmic movement.

10.5.4 In which sequence are the elements experienced?

The necessity really to sense the muscles in the experience of character applies in eurythmy therapy to all the sounds, for vowels just as much as for consonants. It is necessary here to note the sequence in which the elements movement, feeling and character appear during the movement of a sound. In a vowel exercise, the character is regularly emphasized in the finishing position. The character is also intensely experienced in each of the great vowel exercises, when, for instance, the *A* angle of the arms must be maintained through the increasing tempo when swinging the sound.

Before starting to form a vowel, an experienced eurythmist will first call up before their soul the periphery element veil. No movement is yet perceptible through the senses, and yet the whole sound is already present as an inner conception or tableau in the feeling. From this forming of the vowel out of the veil, the eurythmist has the right starting point for the movement; they then let the vowel appear through the movement element. According to the vowel's emphasis of will, the character will already be hinted at during the course of movement; it should always be the dominant aspect when it comes to the ending conformation. There is one exception to this general rule: when it comes to the *Ei*, there is no final position, no arresting of the movement in the character. The elements movement and character alternate in their intensity; the feeling is always around this sound.

When looking at the eurythmy figures, it is not possible to tell when 'character' dominates during the consonant movements. Reflecting on the starting point for this investigation, however, can lead one further: the consonants are developed in the Eurythmy Therapy Course out of a opposite order to that of speech (see Section 6.1). We described how the will element in speech is revealed most clearly in the impactive part of the sound formation. The tensing of the muscles at the onset of speaking the impact sounds *K, T* or *P* can be felt right into the muscles of the abdomen and into the diaphragm. Only afterward does the stream of speech flow on and reveal its movement part. The order is reversed for the eurythmic formation of the consonants: in moving the impact sounds, the movement element dominates at first; the formed sound ends with a final position in the character. The muscles are supposed to be felt in eurythmy therapy. When fast movements take place, character is already present during the course of the activity, becoming dominant at the end. Eurythmic forming of the impact sounds ends with the emphasis on character. Some experienced eurythmists can even describe the starting point for forming the impact sounds, which has to be taken hold of before any movement is visible. They say that character is already within this preparatory tableau of the sound. The question as to the point in time when the veil element should be incorporated is left open as far as this observation is concerned.

It is the other way round with the blown sounds: speaking the *H* begins by blowing strongly; the spoken sound formation ends with a little concluding impact, which contains the character element within itself. In eurythmy, the formation of the blown sounds is again the other way round: the *H* begins with the contracted force of character. The sensation of power predominates here; afterward the stream of movement flows and movement predominates. Eurythmic forming of the blown sounds begins with the emphasis on character.

The element of movement dominates in the preparatory tableau for the blown sounds. Here, too, the time when the veil should be incorporated remains an open question.

It was already stated above for the middle sounds that the blowing and impact elements alternate rapidly, both in speech and in eurythmy. Impacting and moving on freely alternate in speech in rapid succession with these sounds. For all the middle sounds in eurythmy, too, the dominance of movement and character alternates in the shaping of the sounds. The elements movement and character can be kept in a heightened state of balance through a powerful flow of movement.

The middle sounds have to work on the central aspects of the building up processes in the human being. They should give the organism the power to guide the healing processes and substances necessary for building up to those places which have become ill. In this regard, it is particularly important that the character works strongly.

Descriptions as to which element predominates for the middle sounds in the preparatory tableau vary widely.

In conducting the exercise, the eurythmy therapist must take hold of the sequence of movement, feeling and character so consciously that the patient unconsciously imitates this ordering and can sense the character as muscular tension in themselves, without having their attention drawn to it.

The elements movement, feeling and character have not so far been described in connection with those aspects of the soul exercises that do not appear as sounds (affirming/denying, sympathy/antipathy, love/hope, laughter/veneration).

10.5.5   Summary

In preparing the formation of a sound, the appropriate mood of the sound is developed. This contains in a kind of tableau the seeds of all three elements: movement, feeling and character.

In the vowels and impact sounds, the movement is accomplished first; then follows the character, dominating at the end. In the blown sounds, the character is first grasped, only then does the movement element come to the fore. With the middle sounds and the *Ei*, the elements movement and character alternate rhythmically. The elements movement and character are in each case intensified in the transformation of eurythmy to eurythmy therapy; feeling recedes into the background.

11. Harmonizing Speaking and Moving

11.1 When does the therapist speak and when does the patient move?

We saw in Chapter 6 that the eurythmic movement of the consonants develops out of the transformation of the movement of speech. This manifests in the forming of the more blown, flowing aspects of speech, as well as in its more impacting and contracting aspects. In speech, the impact sounds begin with the impactive element, while with the blown sounds the ending is impactive. This order is reversed in eurythmy: here the movement comes at the beginning of the formation of impact sounds and at the end of the movement of the blown sounds. The impactive element in speech is called character in eurythmy; blowing becomes movement.

For all consonants, the sequence of the flowing and the impactive elements is reversed when going from speech to eurythmy.

Speech sequence of impact sounds:
    Beginning: impactive   End: blowing
Eurythmy sequence of impact sounds:
    Beginning: moving   End: emphasizing character

Speech sequence of blown sounds:
    Beginning: blowing   End: impactive
Eurythmy sequence of blown sounds:
    Beginning: emphasizing character End: moving

With all vowels, speech begins – after a tiny little click (aleph) – with movement, and finishes with a very definite ending, brought about either by a succeeding consonant or by an impact-like termination of the airflow.

The eurythmy movement of the vowels begins with movement and ends with character.

The classic structure of the eurythmy therapy exercise was described in more detail in the previous chapter 10. We shall now explore the timing of the speaking of the consonant by the therapist and the movement by the patient.

The following holds good for the impact sounds: the onset of speech is pent up to start with and not yet audible. During this time, the eurythmic gesture begins to flow: the movement becomes visible before the sound is heard, it is anticipated. The eurythmy movement then appears simultaneously with the still inaudible, impactive character of speech. Then as the impact sound becomes audible, the movement aspect of speech predominates. During this flowing sounding of the speech, the ending position is reached, in which muscular tension appears in the eurythmic movement. The movement element of the speech sounds at the same time as the eurythmic character is expressed.

The opposite order applies to the blown sounds, if we pay attention to the exact timing of speech and eurythmic movement. With the blown sounds, the onset of speech begins blowing and flowing. Simultaneously, eurythmic gesture should manifest in the concentrated gesture, emphasizing character at the beginning of the gesture. When the speech then finishes the blown sound with a delicate impact, the eurythmy movement aspect unfolds. With the blown sounds, the eurythmic movement follows the speech; it does not anticipate, as with the impact sounds.

The middle sounds are in between once more. The spoken sound now resounds, with its alternation of impactive and blowing parts, simultaneously with the eurythmy, which alternates between movement and character.

The precise order should be known, so that when working with patients there can be freedom to diverge in particular cases.

11.2 The danger of speaking while demonstrating eurythmy

We have had many opportunities to observe eurythmists and eurythmy therapists, and would like to point to a danger. Regardless of whether in eurythmy therapy or in evening classes, we have again and again observed colleagues simultaneously speaking and moving eurythmically.

Let us go back to basics. The whole human finds expression in the movement of the speech organs. During speech, a wholeness of conceptual content, feelings and impulses of will is summoned up out of a germinal state by the human being. The speech organism is moved in all its parts by the ether body, in such a way that speech is an expression both of the personality and of the content that needs to be expressed. When you do eurythmy, the ether body has to undertake the same activity simultaneously in the limbs. When speaking and movement happen at the same time, the ether body has to do opposite things simultaneously in two different places, for 'the eurythmic element has to stand as polar opposite to the actual process of speech' (p. 32). This dual, opposing activity damages the ether body if done simultaneously.

This can be further elucidated by an example: the ether body, during the day, is active in the human being of nerves and senses in such a way that thoughts can be formed. Forming thoughts is accompanied by a gradual breaking down of the nerves. During the night, it cannot let any thoughts arise; instead the brain is regenerated once more. The ether body cannot simultaneously sustain while building up, and form thoughts while breaking down. In the same way, it cannot simultaneously form the sound in speech and in the limbs. We should not demand the identical activity of the ether body simultaneously on different levels of the threefold human being. The day side and the night side of its activity should not be intermingled. The ether body is damaged and weakened when speaking and doing eurythmy at the same time. We may rapidly alternate between speaking and doing; it is only *simultaneous* opposing activities that have an ill effect.

12. The Spatial Relationships

12.1 The direction of eurythmy therapeutic movement

There is only one place in the Course where an indication appears concerning the relationship of the location where speech is formed in the mouth and the predominant direction of the eurythmic gesture. 'And when you want to express the other element, you can express the labial *R* by carrying the movement further downwards; the lingual *R* can be made more in the horizontal, and the palatal *R* rather more upwards' (pp. 33f). It is striking that here too forming speech and moving are opposite: the palate sounds formed far down should be expressed upward; the lip sounds formed far up should be expressed in a downward direction.

While this statement relates only to the *R*, a general rule suggests itself whereby the eurythmy therapeutic effect is enhanced.

1. Lip sounds are typically directed downward as movement.
2. Teeth sounds are typically shaped horizontally as movement.
3. Palate sounds are typically formed upward as eurythmic movement.

This rule is suggested for eurythmy therapy only.

12.2 The locations of movement and of the effect

The relationship of the location of the illness to the place of therapeutic activity should also be examined. It will be remembered that in physiotherapy (Section 5.1) the location of the illness and the place of therapeutic intervention are generally close together. In a painful case of lumbago, the therapeutic aim will be to release the block by active and passive means and restore normal mobility. Movement therapy can begin peripherally, but will approach the location of the block itself as soon as possible.

In eurythmy therapy, several examples point to the conclusion that this simple relation between the main location of an illness and the therapeutic intervention does not hold true. In the fifth lecture, three spatial relationships of illness to therapeutic measures are described, one after the other.

Because these examples appear in the Eurythmy Therapy Course close to the soul exercises, some eurythmists regard them as soul exercises (see Chapter 9), even though they have a totally different gesture.

12.2.1 Migraine – B

This type of *B* should mainly be deployed for migraine. The location of the pain does not move; the place where the therapy is effective is in the legs: migraine or other headaches should be healed with an exercise which particularly emphasizes bending and stretching movements of the legs. In migraine, substances which have not yet been sufficiently refined rise in an unhealthy way into the building up processes in the head. The pain of migraine is the organism's attempt to overcome this inner poisoning. How the *B* works therapeutically was described in Section 6.2.3: the force in the organism, through which substances are qualitatively transformed and refined should be enhanced. They can work in the head properly only when they have reached the level of quality where they are open to the self, the I.

12.2.2 Irregularities in the abdomen – M

This exercise described immediately following the migraine–*B*, is the opposite. The patient with irregularities in the abdomen – painful dysmenorrhea – should form the *M* with her head. Care must be taken that the head makes a purely right-to-left movement in shaping the *M*. Turning would go against the movement of *M*. The *M* is made simultaneously in the middle region, also with the arms. Again a symptom of illness below is healed through the therapy's being applied at the opposite pole, above. It was suggested in Section 6.2.4 that the *M* should be applied for illnesses where the time processes of the organ-building ether body have fallen into disorder. This is confirmed by the indication: the course of the menstrual period is regulated through the *M*.

12.2.3 Ordering the rhythm of breathing and circulation – R

Influencing the rhythms of breathing and circulation should be undertaken with the *R*. This group of illnesses is situated in the middle region of the body, and the eurythmy gestures should be applied in the middle. The rule in Section 12.2 is confirmed here: it is important at which level of the body the eurythmy exercises are done for the different consonants and in which direction.

The order of the descriptions points again to a rule: eurythmy therapy is applied in the opposite location; migraine is treated through movements of the legs, complaints in the abdomen through movements of the head. The further apart the locations of the ailment and the intervention are, the surer we can be that the therapy is working on the ether body. Physiotherapy looks for the site of the disorder and implements the therapy locally. Identity of the location of the illness and the place where the therapy takes effect can be termed physical. Eurythmy therapy is a therapy where self-regulation is stimulated and which is effective indirectly – according to the laws of the ether body – from the polar opposite location.

13. Embryological Formative Gestures and their Reflection in Eurythmy Therapy

13.1 The spiritual forces of becoming

The lecture of April 18, 1921 forms the high point and conclusion of the Second Medical course (*Anthroposophical Spiritual Science and Medical Therapy*) on the one hand, and of the Eurythmy Therapy Course, on the other. The conceptual content of both courses is aimed toward this joint finale. The beginning of this lecture reaches far back into the past: into a time in which the evolution of the earth and that of the human being were closely linked. It is indicated that three creative forces interacted at that time in the configuration of the earth organism and of the human body. As far as the forming of the earth is concerned, these forces have almost completely ceased working. During embryonic development they still work in the microcosm in forming the body. They are described in this function as follows.

13.1.1 The formative forces

The forming, shaping formative forces are named. They are active everywhere and take hold of the germinating point of a developing organ, The eye is taken as an example. The centripetal forming of the lens from the embryonic skin, on one hand, and the centrifugal evagination of elements of the brain into the inner part of the eye, on the other, are vivid examples of these shaping, formative forces. The description links on to that in the first eurythmy therapy lecture, where the formative impulses of the larynx and the back of the head are brought into relationship with one another. These shaping, form-giving forces and their connection with the zodiac are described in more detail in the lecture 'The Forming of Man through Cosmic Influences.'[1]

13.1.2 The secreting forces

No formative, shaping impulse, intervening for the first time, can be effective if it does not meet the growing point; this contains living substances which are capable of development and, later, of being formed. The fertilized human egg with all its layers and substances is open to be shaped. Other examples are the areas of embryonic skin that become the lens, or the parts of the embryonic nervous system that are formed into the retina. All these germinating points must be receptive for the new formative impulses. Not every place in the developing embryo is open for formative impulses which can lead to the beginnings of new organs. This receptivity is often accomplished by the most minute quantities of substances being eliminated from cells in certain patterns. This makes possible the transformation of a skin cell into a lens cell or the development of an area of the brain into the retina. The formative forces can only become effective and allow new forms to come into existence if, at the same time, traces of substances – calcium has been the most researched of these[2] – are secreted from the cell and work back into the cell membrane.

A corresponding process can also be observed in the adult organism. For every growth and every process of regeneration, the corresponding cytokines and hormones are needed. These must be eliminated in order to make the cells receptive for formative processes and for healing. All secretions into the blood as excretions or hormones, and into the cells as cytokines, serve the life processes of the organism. The minute building blocks described by science complement the results of anthroposophy. The formative forces work from the periphery of the cosmos. They become effective only if they meet processes of secretion. These processes are the second of the forces of becoming described in the lecture.

Steiner describes secretion as a middle life-process in lectures and in *Anthroposophy, a Fragment*. This life process describes the preparation and working of substances for specialized functions, whether they be excretes, hormones or cytokines. As the polar opposite to this process of elimination, Steiner describes how substances have to be qualified for the different levels of existence. They have to be 'secreted upward, aloft' from a more mineralized to a living and soul-bearing quality, until finally they are able to serve the self, the I, of the human being. This upward-tending secretion process of inner potentizing has been described by Steiner and has been explained in detail as a physiological process.[3] This ascending metamorphosis of substance is only possible if the polar opposite, balancing gestures occur: substances become more specialized and gradually more 'foreign,' because they have been eliminated. They then serve from outside as an instrument of many physiological processes.

This aspect of the life process of secretion was presented in the description of the lip sounds *B* and *F* (Section 6.2.3) and the vowel *A* (Section 7.3.3).

This central life process of elimination or secretion is referred to in the seventh lecture on eurythmy therapy. The sevenfold stages of quality of the eliminated substances are characterized and differentiated as 'stages of life' in the lectures of 1921 on 'The Forming of Man through Cosmic Influences.'[4]

13.1.3 The anchoring or consolidation forces

The force of anchoring (or consolidation*) is mentioned in the seventh lecture as a third necessary force during the embryonic development of organs. Anchoring describes a process whereby a previously active, moving object becomes fixed. This third force is also to be observed in embryonic development: all embryonic organs show movement during growth. The organs take a longer or shorter route to their destined place. This movement must come to rest (except in the case of white blood corpuscles and sperm cells) before an organ can function. One can look at the same examples: in the development of the eye, the rudimentary lens is formed on the surface and moves inward. The corresponding parts of the brain grow and move outwards toward the lens. The blood vessels grow and move into the eye socket and the optic nerve grows backwards from the retina into the brain. We are not accustomed to describing these changes as movement. These are subtle, gradual movements that are caused not by muscles, but by growth. They show a sequence with a beginning and an end, which is here called 'anchoring.' If the growth movements do not come to an end, or end too soon, the eyeball – in the example given – will be too large or too small, or other malformations will arise. The concept of anchoring, which Steiner uses here, describes just the end of a hidden movement.

The eye, which is taken in the lecture as an example, enables perception only after its correct development. The function of the eye is perception. Every wrong acting of the shaping, secreting or moving/anchoring forces leads to a malformation of the eye or at least to a diminishing of the eyesight. The same goes for all organs: the forces of becoming – shaping, secreting and moving/anchoring – must act in the right way during organ development, so that the organ can be formed and then serve the soul-spiritual nature of the human being.

* 'Consolidation' is often used in English translations, but it does not properly express the meaning of the German *befestigen* which means to fix down or anchor. Consolidation is closer to the German *verfestigen*.

13.2 The transformation of forces of becoming into living processes

The pre-birthly, spiritual formative forces initiate processes in the ether body which lead to the process of building form. Examining this process of forming, we find the well-known duality of all living processes. Two processes work together to form the eye: on the one hand, activating growth processes on the other, a process of monitoring and holding in check takes place at every step. This holds good for every process of organ formation: life processes of growth and dying work together to give the specific shape and function of an organ. For instance, there are many blood vessels in the eye socket during its development that die off long before birth, in order that the eye can perceive. In the process of development the whole organism as well as every part shows death processes (apoptoses) working together with forces of growth. Before birth, both forces are still working out of the cosmos, from the periphery. Later they manifest in the upper and lower processes which work together everywhere in their regulated, ordered way (Chapter 2).

The same wholeness, regulated in this polar fashion, must also be taken into account when examining the process of elimination/secretion. Here too the building up, lower forces of the human ether body are more active in the creation of substances which are to be secretions; while the breaking down, upper forces are more active in the structure of how the process of elimination is started.

In the same way, the force of moving/anchoring is active out of its duality in spatial and chronological ordering and regulating. The interplay of the processes of the upper and lower human being is everywhere the basis for development, for the work of the ether body. The three forces named in this lecture originate in a sphere which is higher spiritually than the etheric forces; they originate from the astral sphere. From this sphere, they set in motion the processes of forming and shaping, of elimination, and of the movements of life. The course of each process unfolds out of the laws of the ether body, described with the concepts of the upper and lower human being.

All organs in the human body are formed through the interplay of three primal forces. The three formative forces are still active when the organs are completed, and manifest in the function of the organ, in its processes of building up and breaking down. The formative, secretory and movement/anchoring forces come into effect in the field of tension of the upper and lower human being.

13.3 The three forces as capacities of soul

The three basic forces, here called formative force, secretion and moving/ anchoring, work mainly until an organ has reached functional maturity. They work together in all the organs in order to form them to be capable of functioning.

The pre-birthly, spiritual, formative forces work out of the widths of the cosmos. They descend and transform themselves into processes of the ether body, manifesting in the upper and lower organization. There they shape the building up processes of all organ formation during the embryonic phase. The lecture refers to the goal of the embryonic development of the eye: perception. Only after birth does the eye open and take on the function of perception, long after its formation has been completed. The soul and spirit can now use the body; the eye serves sight. The human being is born with the potential for sight. When the child begins to perceive in a differentiated manner, the next process of soul can awaken. The formative forces transform into the activity of *thinking*. The formative function which comes to expression here corresponds to the upper forces. They effect the breaking down processes (Table 1, page 20).

The other pre-birthly forces work through the earth in an opposite direction as the formative forces. The spiritual forces of moving/ anchoring appear during embryonic development in the ability of the ether body to move cells, tissues and even organs to the place where they are to function. Again, the upper and lower forces act together. These movement/ anchoring forces appear as *will* when active in the soul. They are more closely connected with the building up, lower forces than with the upper forces.

The spiritual secretory forces descend in the same way from the astral sphere and appear in the living processes for building secretions and for elimination. This field of tension is another revelation of the upper and lower human being. The building up and breaking down forces are in a balanced relationship in the secretion process. These etheric forces appear in the soul as *feeling* (Section 4.1.2).

13.4 Metamorphosis of the three forces into spiritual capacities

These three forces are further described in the seventh lecture. They should be actively transformed in the human soul into spiritual activity. Then thinking becomes the faculty of *intuition*. In the same way, through following a path of spiritual development, the spiritual capacity of secretion which has taken part in building the body and which has been liberated in the soul as feeling, can be developed into *inspiration*. The spiritual force of moving/anchoring, which has created the inner order of the body, reveals its activity within the soul as will and can be further developed into the power of *imagination*.

spiritual force	*soul activity*	*spiritual capacity*
formative forces	thinking	intuition
secretion	feeling	inspiration
anchoring	will	imagination

13.5 The three forces and the organism in eurythmy therapy

In the first six lectures, the vowel and consonant forces of speech and their metamorphosis into the healing sound movements are described. Eurythmy therapy is based on these processes of transformation. In the seventh lecture the macrocosmic aspect is added. The three active spiritual forces – formative forces, forces of secretion and forces of movement/anchoring – are elements of the creative world of the logos. They become threefold living processes which unfold in the ether body in the reciprocal activity of upper and lower processes. The consonantal and vocalic exercises of eurythmy therapy engage with these reciprocal activities (Figure 8).

This fourfold order arose out of the first six lectures:

— Sounds which work on *movement:*
— The consonants *K, G* and *H* give the force of movement;
— The vowels *I* and *U* give the shape of movement (Section 8.1).

— Sounds which influence *secretion* and specialized substances:
— The consonants *T, D, S* and *Sh* support the forming of substances for special functions;
— The vowels *O* and *E* effect the distribution of secretions (Section 8.2).

Vowels strengthen the forces of the upper human being

I & U	O & E	A	Ei* & Au*
Not being able to stand/walk. Being able to begin and end movement and repose.	Being too fat or too thin. Being able to begin and end the forming of functional substance.	Being able to overcome animal nature. Being able to transform individualized substances to a quality that can bear the self or I.	Being able to mediate form-impulses out of the cosmos and the earth for the human form. * Not mentioned in the Course
Movement and rest: consolidation	**Processes of elimination enable the building of human substance**		**Formative forces shape organs**
Having strength for movement	Being able to build up functional substance	Enabling substances to become capable of transformation to self or I quality	Substances can take up impulses of form
K & H	**D & S**	**B & F**	**M/N L R**

Consonants strengthen the forces of the lower human being

Figure 8: The connection of the vowel and consonant exercises with the three embryological developmental gestures

— Sounds which influence the *transformation of substance*:
— The consonants *B* and *F* mediate the force of transformation of substances and their potentization to an individualized quality;
— The vowel *A* orders the steps of qualitative development to a higher level (Section 8.3).

— Sounds which influence the individuation of organs and their specific substances
— The consonants *M, N, L* and *R* provide the welling power of becoming;
— The vowels *Au* and *Ei* form the shaping (Section 8.4).

This fourfold ordering of the influences of the vowels and consonants, which arises from the first six lectures of the Eurythmy Therapy Course, is condensed in the seventh lecture into a threefold ordering. Viewed methodologically, it is the same step of transformation which is necessary to proceed from an insight into the fourfold ordering of living processes

– in the lecture, 'The Invisible Human Being Within Us,'[5] they are called the systems of nerves, respiration, circulation and metabolism – to an understanding of the threefolding of the human organism. The perspective moves from the plane in which living development takes place to the order within the world of soul. The system of nerves and senses, that of metabolism and the limbs and, between them, the rhythmic system now appear. The human soul forces of thinking, feeling and the will use the organism which is itself formed in a threefold manner. The cosmic, pre-birthly forces of thinking, feeling and the will created the preconditions for this, when the forces of becoming were transformed into living functions. For this reason, the two middle processes of the fourfold ordering – the externalized secretions and the internalized transformation of substances – are summarized in the seventh lecture. The two functional processes are part of what is called the life process of secretion in the seventh lecture (see Section 13.1, section 2).

The three fundamental cosmic forces – formative forces, forces of secretion, and anchoring – can be ordered anew through vowel and consonant eurythmy therapy where an illness or a malfunction has developed. The forces of movement and anchoring, which correspond to the ordering of the will and the building up processes, can be connected to the consonants. The forces of secretion, which unfold in the alternation of building up and breaking down, are related to the vowels; and the formative forces with the working together of vowel and consonant.

Most eurythmy therapeutic exercises are built up of vowels and consonants, and so all three forces can be activated specifically. When a particular illness or pathological function needs to be influenced it is good to draw on the corresponding processes with their vowel and consonant elements.

The eurythmy therapist practises the healing sounds with the patient. The sounds initially make an imprint into the whole organism through breaking down processes specific to the particular sound. During sleep, the cosmic archetype is impressed into the vital body. Steiner liked to take the image of a footprint in the snow as a picture of such an imprint. After the exercise, during the short rest afterwards, the cosmic forces orient themselves on the imprint and work therapeutically. Of course, this presupposes that the sounds have been impressed deeply enough into all the malfunctioning organs.

In the seventh lecture, which begins with the cosmic past of the human being, there is the following important prediction:

> People in the future will in general tend to be deformed in the most manifold ways, because they will no longer be able to build up the normalizing human form out of the involuntary active forces The

human being will become free even in respect to the building up of their own form. (p. 97)

The 'involuntary active forces' – the formative forces, the forces of secretion and those of movement and anchoring – will in future less and less be able to have an effect out of themselves. They must now be understood and taken hold of by human beings, in order to enable healthy bodily development into the future. Eurythmy and eurythmy therapy have the task consciously to impress these 'involuntary active forces' bodily into the human being; so that the formative forces, the processes of secretion and the forces of moving/anchoring can work in future in such a way that the formation of the human being can continue to remain effective, whole and unscathed.

14. Examples of Therapeutic Words

In this chapter, some eurythmy therapy exercises which originated with Rudolf Steiner will be examined to see whether the proposed systematization is confirmed or whether there are contradictions. These exercises are a sequence of vowels and consonants and are sometimes called 'therapeutic words.' The indications about the patients and the exercises undertaken are from Margarete Kirchner-Bockholt's book. The connection of the illness to the eurythmy therapy prescribed has not been checked in every case. The cancer sequence is examined first, as our work together started with this. An understanding of the pathological processes of cancer and its transformation through the different therapies makes it necessary to grasp this therapeutic 'word' ever anew.

14.1 The cancer sequence $O-E-M-L-Ei-B-D$

The origin of this exercise is described in Kirchner-Bockholt's book: the cancer sequence was recommended for a 32-year-old, English-speaking patient 'who had been operated on and afterwards had undergone radiation treatment for cancer of the breast.' It is unclear whether an *Ei* (as in 'bite') or an *I* (as in 'beet') was recommended.

In cases of cancer, malignant tissue growths develop from surface tissues. In these – as everywhere – there is normally a balance, specific to the organ, between impulses which foster growth and those which inhibit it. Oncogenes and tumor suppressor genes are the molecular tools which, in cancer, are no longer integrated into the organism as a whole. Both processes become independent and secrete substances. On the one hand, there is a hyperfunction of signals which ought to inhibit. Because they are faulty, however, they are unable to take effect. At the same time, the stimuli which promote growth are too strong. Through this overactivity of the upper and lower processes, the cancer cells attain a relative degree of permanence; they canot die. The shaping formative forces, the processes of secretion, and (in metastasis) also the forces of moving/anchoring are increasingly altered pathologically. A fuller description of cancer from the aspect of the upper and lower processes can be found elsewhere.[1]

The illness progresses from a microcarcinoma, that shows hardly any tendency to growth, to an invasive growth which destroys the neighbouring organs; and later spreads in metastases through active cell movement. If no therapeutic intervention occurs, cancer normally progresses and leads slowly to death. Spontaneous recovery is extremely rare.

The pathological secretion processes which led to the unbridled growth should be normalized through the vowels *O* and *E* and the corresponding *D*. In addition, *B* supports the force which builds up individualized substances. The force in the organism which deals with organ-specific shaping and forming should be strengthened with *M*, *L* and *Ei*.

It is striking that the series contains no blown sounds on the one hand, and no movement sounds (*G* & *H* and *I* & *U*) on the other. Impact sounds predominate, perhaps because the pathological event begins deep in the centre of the cell's metabolism, regardless of where the tumour is located. The movement sounds may be introduced additionally if metastases are confirmed. This stage of the illness arises because cancer cells, besides their unbridled growth, regain the embryonal capacity to migrate actively. The *U* is helpful in this phase.

14.2 Chronic constipation, meteorism *L–T / D–R*

Besides constipation and flatulence, a disposition to cancer has also been described.[2] This disposition is based on the findings of image analysis, like sensitive crystallization, capillary dynamolisis, etc., rather than on clinical diagnosis.

The secretion sounds *T* & *D* are in the centre of the exercise; the formation of intestinal secretions should be stimulated. A general activation of the building up forces through the middle sounds *R* and *L* should also happen.

A striking feature is the doubling up of the therapy with *T* plus *D*. Other patients have received similar doublings up (*G* plus *K*, *B* plus *P*). The therapeutic significance of this is not in evidence in the Course, and is also not established in Kirchner-Bockholt's work. This doubling up is also surprising, because in the fourth lecture a qualitatively similar effect is elaborated: 'when one carries out what we call the soft sound, one can remedy milder conditions; with what we call the hard sound, more severe [acute] conditions of this sort' (pp. 47f). That is, the harder impact or blown sounds work more strongly on the illness or the symptoms.

14.3 A child with hemiplegia S–M–A / L–M–Y / T–M–U

This four-year-old child is presented extensively as the fourth case in the book *Extending Medical Practice* by Steiner & Wegman. The aim of the therapy is described: the I-organization of the child should be stimulated in such a way that the astral body becomes livelier and its affinity with the ether body is increased. Kirchner-Bockholt describes the different exercises in her Chapter 12. The middle sound *M* stands in the centre here. Through it, the child's development and the proper forming of organs can be promoted. For this, a qualitative refinement of substances – through the *A* – is required. Above and beyond that, the therapy with *A* aims at an intensified transformation of the child's inherited body. Secretion processes are stimulated through the *S* at the beginning and the *T* in the last stage of the exercise. The *U* is possibly there for the treatment of motor restlessness in the paralysed side. In the concluding evaluation it was said that the child had become calmer and more agile: 'the excess of clumsy movement has declined.' It is puzzling that a *Y* [German *J*] was chosen for the exercise and not the *I*.

14.4 Teething problems in the upper jaw L–A, and the lower jaw L–O

This sequence was introduced in the Stuttgart lecture. Misalignments of individual teeth in the dental arch are what is probably meant. The *L* fits well into the systematization attempted here: as a key building up sound it promotes organ formation. The directional indications which Steiner describes are puzzling: 'In the case of the upper teeth, the sculptural activity that forms them is active from the front backwards ... In the teeth of the lower jaw the sculptural activity works from the back to the front.' (p. 113). Even after consulting with orthodontists it has so far not been possible to discover the phenomenon referred to. The plastic, shaping activity refers here to the formative upper forces. The dynamic of growth of the teeth is easy to observe: the enamel part of each of the upper teeth is formed and finished within the upper jaw; it only has to be moved from above downward; the enamel parts of the teeth in the lower jaw have to be moved from below upward. This movement takes place in a complex spiralling way. But what is meant by 'from the front backwards'? The different effects of *A* and *O* have not yet been clarified for this context.

14.5 Motor restlessness, fidgeting *L−U−O−K−M*

In Chapter 12 of her book, Kirchner-Bockholt refers to 'a boy with motor restlessness and fidgeting': both the *U* and the *K*, which were prescribed, fit well into the ordering of the indications we propose. The rhythm of moving and resting should be regulated with vowels and consonants. A general building up should be achieved through the middle sounds *L* and *M*. Only the allocation of the *O* remains unclear owing to the sparse descriptions of the boy and his illness.

14.6 Dementia *R−L−S−I*

This child is described at length in the Curative Education Course.[3] Central to the illness is that certain proteins in the metabolism had not been sufficiently structured with sulphur when they were being built up. In the case of this child, the breaking down of nutrition was stimulated therapeutically through the *S*. The building up of protein in the body can only happen when the breaking down of foreign protein has happened in the right way. Two middle sounds were also recommended, in order to promote the ether body's activity of organ formation in the body. The symptoms appeared 'because the conscious life of soul is up there, but down below the unconscious is unrestrained.' The vowel *I* fits into this description: unconscious lower processes should be brought into movement and regulated. Kirchner-Bockholt describes the child very briefly in her Chapter 12.

14.7 Disorder of the liver and intestine, dysphylaxia, cold feet *L I − M A − R U*

The patient is a 48-year-old woman with a disorder of the liver and intestine, interrupted sleep and cold feet.[4] The description of the illness reminds one of the references in connection with the 'too-weak intervention' of the higher human sheaths.[5] All the middle sounds are called on in this sequence. In addition, the patient should better be able to enter into internal and external movement processes through doing the *I* and *U* together. She should enhance the building up of her organs with the middle sounds, after the production of substance has been structured in the *A*.

14.8 Hypothyroidism $S-M-I-A$

Steiner is said to have diagnosed 'a hypotension and hypertonia of the thyroid' in this patient, 'a case of Graves' disease which was not fully developed.'[6] It was said that she was small, pale, bloated, myxedematous and tired quickly. There was also stiffness in the legs and flatulence. Walking was to be enhanced with the vowel *I*; gastro-intestinal secretion for breaking down nutrition stimulated with the *S*, which should also stimulate the thyroid's eliminatory function. The *A* should activate the building up of individualized substance. *M*, as a middle sound, enables the building up of the organs once more.

14.9 Hay fever $T-S-R-M-A$

Apart from hay fever, the patient suffered also from pains in the nerves and muscles, headaches and a weak bladder.[7] With hay fever, the foreignness of substances in the environment cannot be properly 'digested.' The symptoms are characterized by too much secretion of nasal mucous and tears. As middle sounds, *R* and *M* have to activate the building up of organs. *T* and *S* point to ordering anew the secretion in the intestine and in the nasal passage. The patient's formation of individualized substance should be strengthened with the *A*.

14.10 Conclusion

Some of the sound sequences suggested by Steiner have been examined to see whether the sounds recommended become more comprehensible through the ordering of the indications presented here. Unfortunately, the indications on the patients and their illnesses are so fragmentary that an assessment of the patient's condition and an evaluation of the differential diagnosis are not possible. It is striking that many middle sounds are used. The other sounds used can also mostly be allocated meaningfully. To that extent, it is helpful to look at the historical examples together with the order of indications presented here. But it is an open question whether one would choose the same sounds today.

15. Future Tasks of Physicians and Eurythmy Therapists

An important problem in the development of eurythmy therapy up till now is that there is hardly a common language between physicians and eurythmy therapists. Medical diagnoses these days are defined by concepts based on molecular biology and from details arising out of differential diagnosis. Understanding is further impeded because the translation of scientific diagnoses into a spiritualized language has not yet sufficiently been worked out for many illnesses. The physician thinks and speaks in a jargon which is far removed from any general level of understanding. Their indications for eurythmy therapy are frequently made in the daily stress of the ward or the surgery. Time for reflection or for a conversation with the eurythmy therapist is rarely found.

On the other hand, eurythmy therapy is based on an artistic training, while the basic medical training is often inadequate. Only in recent years has there been a curriculum for training eurythmy therapists, so that a working knowledge of therapeutic procedure in the whole of medicine, in curative education and educational learning support can be acquired. The necessity of an improvement in medical and therapeutic training for the further development of eurythmy therapy has been recognized.

The further development of eurythmy therapy has been hampered by the fact that past experience and therapeutic success have received hardly any publicity. The reports that are available describe various individual experiences. They are couched in general terms and characterize separate events. They generally do not go into why particular sounds were chosen. Written records of individual experiences are a necessary first step. A scientific treatment of eurythmy therapy and a clarification of the connection between a sequence of exercises and a successful treatment require the systematic overview of indications.

At the beginning of the Stuttgart lecture Steiner particularly empha sizes that the basics of eurythmy therapy have been presented in sufficient detail in the course. 'Basically, the empirical material relating to eurythmy therapy was developed and presented in the recent lecture course for physicians in Dornach, and it is hardly necessary to go beyond what was given at that time (p. 106). He calls for an elaboration of the 'physiology of eurythmy therapy.' The Eurythmy Therapy Course – as was stated in Chapter 2 – builds on an understanding of the life processes which develop in the field of tension between the upper and lower human being. The ether body manifests in these upper and lower centres of forces working simultaneously. All four parts of the human being are active in both centres; the vital processes unfold between them in time and space.

In the present work, we have attempted to distil out of the Eurythmy Therapy Course an initial systematic overview with points of reference for ordering and organizing typical processes. We hope that the communication between physicians and eurythmy therapists can be developed further on this basis, and now put forward various suggestions.

15.1 Movement diagnosis by the eurythmist

To help understanding between physician and eurythmy therapist, the eurythmy therapist must first diagnose the patient's movements, following structured guidelines. The diagnosis should always be done with the same exercises for each patient, for instance the three mentioned below. Evaluating eurythmy by the elements of movement, feeling and character is also important. Another aspect of this diagnosis would be whether the approach to movement as a whole is oriented more to vowels or to consonants.

Exercises often used for movement diagnosis include:
1. Contraction and expansion
2. Stepping (forward and backward, in a triangle where appropriate)
3. *I–A–O*

15.2 Questions from the eurythmy therapist to the physician

If there is a prescription for eurythmy therapy, the diagnosis and the age of the patient is recorded there. The possible duration of the treatment will also be known well enough from the situation. There are very different, general guiding principles for the structuring of eurythmy therapy in schools, rehabilitation centres and in hospitals. So the therapist generally knows what cycle of treatment is required. It is usually the case today that the physician does not recommend any sounds for the patient. In this situation, eurythmy therapists have developed many and varied strategies for designing a therapy plan. The following suggestions for questions to put to the physician should help keep their bearings on the Eurythmy Therapy Course.

15.2.1 Questions about the diagnosis

A tabular summary of questions to do with the quality of processes has been compiled below. They relate to the physiology of eurythmy which was established in the Eurythmy Therapy Course. The physicians may not be able to answer the questions quickly. They are used to evaluating the symptoms and taking the etiology, that is the underlying origins of the illness, into their thinking and action. They have less practice in describing the vital processes in which illnesses develop and which lead to the symptoms.

An example can help clarify the matter. The etiology of lung cancer can be sought in the personal makeup of the smoker and in the damage occasioned by the poisons. The symptoms of the illness are, for example, coughing and shortness of breath. The processes driving the growth of the cancer in the organism are revealed in the unbridled enhancement of the lower forces of growth (that is oncogenes) and the equally intensified, but no longer organizing and ordering upper forces (that is tumour suppressor genes). This falling apart of the upper and lower human being should be influenced through the cancer sequence (Section 14.1). The therapy takes its start neither on the level of symptoms nor on that of etiology, for it is the vital processes that are to be influenced.

The procedure will be made easier for the eurythmy therapists if they present the four basic questions to the physician systematically. The answers should give some clues for a therapeutic sequence of sounds. Suggestions can then be listed in the overview as ideas for eurythmy therapeutic exercises. The emphasis and sequence in which the eurythmy therapist builds up the therapeutic 'word' in their work is initially completely open. Nor should their own therapeutic intuition on meeting the patient be constrained. This is an attempt to offer help in looking at the pathological processes in such a way that medical knowledge and experience in movement therapy can work together better.

Knowledge of the processes specific to the illness together with the individual situation of the patient determine the therapeutic course of action.

1. To what extent is the illness based on a pathological muscle activity?
— movement disorders of the voluntary muscles *H*
— movement disorders of the smooth muscles in vessels, bronchi, stomach *H*
— movement disorders of the smooth muscles in the intestine, urogenital tract *G–K*
— displacement on the cellular level (for instance metastasis) *G–K*
— is the flow of movement impaired? *I*
— can repose not be maintained? *U*

2. To what extent is the illness caused by a disorder of secretion formation or of the building up of substances specialized for specific functions?
— secretion disorders of the skin *Sh–S*
— deficiency or excess of secretion, hormones or cytokines, in the areas of the nose, throat or lung? *Sh–S*
— deficiency or excess of secretion, hormones or cytokines, in the gastro-intestinal or urogenital tract? *D–T*
— excess of secretion or of formation of functional and storage substances *O*
— deficiency of secretion or of functional substances? *E*

3. Disorders of the formation of individualized substance
— secretion disorders of the glands *F–V*
— are foreign substances not being properly broken down? (contact allergies, respiratory allergies, nutritional allergies) *F–V*
— do substances become 'foreign' again in the organism, as a secondary effect, in terms of auto-immune processes? *F–V*
— can individualized substances not be sufficiently built up? *B–P*
— is the ordering and supervising of the formation of individualized substance working sufficiently? *A*

4. Disorders in the building up of shape or function of an organ
— an organ is unable to develop its capacity to function, or develops too fast and too far *M*
— an organ loses its relation to the building up night-time processes *L*
— an organ is no longer properly integrated with the vital processes *R*
— the pathologically altered vital processes 'maintenance,' 'growth' and 'reproduction should be ordered in such a way that:
  – cosmic formation can become effective *Ei*
  – earthly formation can become effective *Au*

15.2.2 The patient's life circumstances and mental state

It is important for the eurythmy therapist to know about crucial aspects of the patient's life circumstances and about their mental state, in order not to make mistakes through tactlessness or ignorance. Such knowledge could modify the eurythmy therapy. Eurythmy therapy is a somatic therapy which intends to bring about processes of healing on the level of the ether body. Bentinck points to this when he writes: 'Only when I really manage to keep eurythmy therapy free of any subjective, artistic elements will it be possible for me to achieve anything meaningful with this therapy. Otherwise I would have to be content with an improvement in general health.'[1]

At this point the eurythmy therapist should be advised against being drawn into giving advice on psychological issues, out of their desire to help, and thereby taking on the task of a counsellor or psychologist. They have neither the mandate nor the training for this. Eurythmy therapy aims to bring about healing processes on the level of the ether body.

15.3 Questions from the physician to the eurythmy therapist

Eurythmy therapy should therapeutically order anew the vital processes that have become one-sided and which underlie illness. These need to be described by the physician in such a way that the eurythmist can come to therapeutic insights that are gained mainly from the illness and only to a lesser extent from the particular patient. By the same token, the eurythmy therapist will need to learn to describe the movement disorders they have perceived in the patient in such a way that the physician can find again the vital processes within them. The physician does not usually need a description of the patient's psychological condition (or at most as part of the general picture). They will also know from the patient whether they enjoy the eurythmy therapy, whether they practise independently, and so on. The physician has to accompany the course of the illness and guide the process of its healing. But they have no real perception of how illnesses are expressed in the patient's eurythmy. They need this characterized, which can be based on the experience of movement, feeling and character. A brief description must give the physician a picture of the patient.

1. How is the whole posture of the patient? Are there any movement disabilities (through stroke, deformities of the joints, and so on)?
2. How is the flow of eurythmy which arises out of the interplay of movement, feeling and character? Are there unconscious asymmetries and stereotypes in the movement?

3. What is their unconscious starting point for eurythmy? Is it more from within and so driven from the soul, or more from without, more mechanical? A description such as that a *B* was done too vocalically, like an *O*, or conversely that an *I* was taken hold of too consonantally, from without, would belong here.

4. Does the patient manage to learn and practise new patterns of movement? Or are they stuck in imitation and can only do the sound well if the therapist demonstrates it for them?

The comments the physician would wish for from the eurythmy therapist could also be more specific:

— How succesful is the patient in doing the consonants from without?

— Does the patient manage to direct the vowel from within?

— Does the patient achieve a perception of their muscular tension as the character of the sound?

— Does the patient balance the three elements in the sound, or does a cramped muscular tension (character) or unrestrained flow of movement predominate?

— Does the patient manage to sound the vowel afterward; and practise the inner experience and perception of the consonant?

— Does the patient manage to let go in the rest afterward?

Several questionnaires for the evaluation of eurythmy therapy are available. See the Appendix for details of a questionnaire with questions relating to movement, feeling and character.

Communication will be difficult if the eurythmy therapist describes to the physician what the patient is unable to do, for instance, that they cannot do the *B* or the *O* properly. The physician cannot gain any real experience of their own from negative statements like these. The therapist also puts obstacles in their own way, as it becomes more difficult to gain insights into how the patient's various inabilities can be overcome.

16. Outline of a Physiology
of Eurythmy Therapy

In the sixth lecture of the Eurythmy Therapy Course it is emphasized
again and again that physiology based on the spiritual must be developed
for the further elaboration of eurythmy therapy. 'When wishing to consider the physiology of eurythmy, it is natural to keep the active, moving
human being in view' (p. 81). As if addressing the eurythmy therapists,
Steiner says, ' the essence ... can already be discovered when eurythmy
is carried out purely artistically' and then continues as if addressing the
physicians, 'and the physiology corresponding to it can then be found'
(p. 71). The following was also addressed to the physicians: 'It will be
seen how this sort of study [eurythmy therapy] will quicken the whole of
physiology' (p. 81).

Ordinary physiology describes the vital processes as measurable,
individual processes. In a spiritual scientific description, it is not the individual procedure with its isolated steps that is characterized, but the field
of tension in which a particular event is integrated.

You can study everything offered you by anatomy, physiology
and biology according to this principle, and you will see that only
thus is light shed on the human organization. As long as you do
not distinguish between the upper and the lower ... you will not
be able to understand the human being. For there is a fundamental
difference between all that goes on in the lower activity of
the organization and what goes on in the activity of the upper
organism.[1]

The enlivening or 'quickening of the whole of physiology' can happen
when all the details which have been described scientifically are recognized as pieces of mosaic. They are markers of a process which unfolds
between the two centres of forces of the etheric body: the lower and upper
organization. Regardless of the processes investigated – the sequence of
steps during coagulation of the blood, or the working of the enzymatic
respiratory chain, or the molecular description of cancer development –

everywhere a duality of activating and inhibiting forces is necessary for the regulation of the process. The attempt has been made in Chapter 2 and Table 1 to indicate the criteria of a living physiology which unfolds between the upper and lower human being. It is important here to recognize that the upper processes are activated and strengthened through vocalic eurythmy therapy; the lower, conversely, through consonantal eurythmy therapy.

In the sixth lecture, the physiology of the hearing of speech and its manifestations in the human being are described. During active listening, etheric processes may be observed supersensibly around the limbs. Comparable etheric movements are to be seen during sleep. Those during listening are more intensive than those during sleep. These impulses of movement belonged originally to the vowels and consonants, and have been lost during the course of evolution. This loss is the reason why the speaking of vowels tends to create illnesses, in the same way as listening to consonants leads to one-sidedness.

There then follows a spiritual examination of the effect that occurs when a person takes in, through hearing, the vocalic forces or alternatively those of the consonants. As the concordant impulses of movement which used to arise when listening to (or speaking) vowels have been lost, the limbs during listening now receive unconscious impulses of movement which are not carried out. They become dammed up and cause pathological dysfunction – as was described for *O* and *E*. The symptoms of the disorder lie primarily in the metabolism: with *O* in an increased formation of substance. They then work into the rhythmical in a secondary effect. In a eurythmy therapeutic vowel exercise, the limbs are moved in a manner specific to the vowel, and the sound is impressed into the whole human being. During the ensuing period of sleep, the pathological dysfunction is healed.

The supersensible physiology of listening to consonants is described at greater length. The process may be divided into several steps. When listening predominantly to consonants, imitative movements are held back and artificially stilled; so the will is dammed up in the limbs. The movement I or self is no longer present in the limbs, nor is the night-time I present, as the person is, after all, awake and listening. This disturbed condition is reflected in the system of nerves and senses and appears as an aura around the person. The latter then produces self-will and self-centredness in the soul. The person is inwardly strong and powerful in the metabolism, and aggressive in the life of soul. The weak head-organization, which has developed too slowly, is strengthened and built up through consonantal eurythmy therapy.

In his lectures, Rudolf Steiner describes very different polarities which are important for understanding the connection between vowels and consonants on the one hand, and the corresponding movements on the other. Supersensible and sensory observations are mentioned. Polar relationships are referred to again and again: listening and moving, functions during sleep and when awake, inner and outer changes, primary influences and secondary reactions are all described in the upper and lower human being. This does not make it easy to understand the text. Often only one pole of the polarities is mentioned. It is an important part of this physiology of eurythmy therapy that the polarity of *perception* and *movement* is described.

Descriptions of physiological processes in scientific textbooks are so detailed that their purpose can easily be overlooked. They explain the measurable facts without any connection to the spiritual reality of the human being. The outline of a spiritual physiology is laid down by Steiner in the two courses, the Second Medical and the Eurythmy Therapy Course. Here he always shows forces with their polar opposite, and how together they underlie all living processes. In his time most of the scientific details had not yet been researched. However, the physiological processes known today can always be described from these two aspects: to what extent does a monitoring and inhibiting aspect or the opposite activating and driving one influence the process? This can always be connected with the upper and lower human being. The same process can be viewed in its molecular detail on one hand, and in the etheric dynamics on the other.

For a physiology of living qualities, the manifold fields of forces, which revealed themselves through their polar connections, can be subdivided into three categories, as they were presented in the final eurythmy therapy lecture.

1. How do the formative forces operate, forming the whole and all the parts?
2. How do the secretion processes regulate the relationship between extracellular and intracellular elements in health and illness, enabling an organism to function?
3. Which processes of movement are necessary for the development of the organism as a whole and in all its parts, and how do these come to rest (anchoring) on reaching functional maturity?

Every living process develops out of an initial seed state and unfolds toward its complete manifestation. This development in time, in specific substances, and in a visible form, takes place between the forming, shaping, inhibiting or breaking down forces on the one hand, and the dynamizing, growth-promoting, building up forces, on the other. The forming of the rudiments of an organ, its development up to functional maturity, and finally the changes through usage and ageing, can be observed, at least in an overall view.

In this description of the elements of eurythmy therapy, an attempt has been made carefully to systematize the field of tension in which life unfolds. The difficulty of making a systematic description is highlighted in the medical course. The two poles of the ether body are once more described, this time as 'upper, back' and 'lower, front' forces.

When one understands this in a comprehensive way, and in the way that the 'upper and back' and the 'lower and front human being' exist together and one above the other ... when we observe that properly ... then we have the whole human being before us and can grasp the human ... in its other processes.[2]

The physiology of eurythmy will develop when the polar forces of the ether body become better differentiated and understood. The elaboration presented here is only a first beginning.

17. Epilogue

Eurythmists who work through this material will discover that a systematic, more scientific treatment of eurythmy therapy puts many different aspects in an accessible conceptual context. This overview has not previously been available in this form. Many practical details may be integrated into everyday consciousness. The emphasis of this study is on the description of how the ether body is directed toward the living physical body and how it can be observed in its living, physiological functions. In the Eurythmy Therapy Course, Rudolf Steiner describes this activity of the ether body by taking a circumscribed realm – that of the metabolism. The intention of this study is to look at this partial realm in such a way that the entirety of the ether body becomes visible through it.

This approach also determines the focus on the four lower senses. In the first description of the eurythmic elements, Rudolf Steiner emphasizes the necessity of conscious experience of these elements. Experiences of weight and levity are the basis of the element of movement; feeling develops from the experience of pressure and suction, working from outside; the experience of tensing and relaxing the muscles creates the basis for character. The eurythmic elements movement, feeling and character include higher levels of experience as well; this is only alluded to in the relevant chapters. The activities of the soul and the I of the therapist and the patient during and after the therapeutic exercises have not been part of the investigation. Comparisons with other movement therapies were only undertaken on the level of the primary perceptions.

Results of the first measurements of variability of heart frequencies (the heartbeat/breathing ratio) during eurythmy therapeutic exercises have not been included in the presentation, as the central theme was to come closer to the Eurythmy Therapy Course. But we hope that future experimental research will complement and deepen this approach.

We hope that those eurythmy therapists who put their therapeutic activity at the disposal of this scientific research will ever and again seek the archetypal source of eurythmy therapy in their continuing practice. Only the manifestations of the sounds have been investigated in this book, not their essential nature. The essence of eurythmy therapy can only be experienced through a path of training in anthroposophy and eurythmy.

Appendix

1. Questionnaire on Eurythmy Therapy

There is a questionnaire available from the Havelhöhe Research Institute, Berlin. An English version is downloadable from
www.fih-berlin.de/html/downloads.html

2. Eurythmy Therapy Training Curriculum

Details of eurythmy therapy training curriculum are available from
www.forumhe-medsektion.net/english/train/Training.html
International Council of Eurythmy Therapy Trainers
Medical Section at the Goetheanum
School of Spiritual Science
4143 Dornach
Switzerland

Notes

1. Introduction

1 CW 303, Jan 5, 1922, evening.

2. Processes of Etheric Body

1 CW 277a, Sep 17, 1912.
2 CW 277a, Aug 28, 1913.
3 CW 313, April 11, 1921.
4 CW 312, March 22, 1920.
5 CW 313, April 11, 1921.
6 CW 319, Aug 28, 1923.
7 Laue 2000.
8 Müller-Wiedemann 1997.
9 CW 319, Nov 16, 1923.

3. Polar Effects

1 CW 313, April 16, 1921.
2 CW 313, April 18, 1921.
3 CW 313, April 15, 1921.
4 CW 305, Aug 17, 1922.
5 CW 277, p. 315, Notebook Feb 18, 1923.
6 CW 319, p. 31, Feb 28, 1923.
7 CW 314, p. 191, Jan 1, 1924.
8 CW 317, July 1, 1924.
9 CW 317, July 4, 1924.
10 CW 317, July 6, 1924.
11 CW 317, July 1, 1924.
12 CW 316, Jan 9, 1924.
13 CW 314, p. 208, Jan 2, 1924.
14 CW 316, p. 133, Jan 9, 1924.
15 CW 313, April 13, 1921.
16 CW 313, April 14, 1921.

4. The Three Elements

1 CW 279, Aug 4, 1922.
2 CW 305, Aug 17, 1923.
3 CW 279, Aug 26, 23.
4 CW 300b, March 1, 1923.
5 CW 305, Aug 17, 1923.
6 CW 279, Aug 4, 1922.
7 CW 279, Aug 4, 1922.
8 CW 170, Aug 15, 1916.
9 Göbel 1982.
10 CW 170, Aug 15, 1916.
11 CW 300b March 1, 1923.
12 CW 303, Jan 5, 1923, in the evening.
13 Parr.

5. Other Movement Therapies

1 CW 300b, March 1, 1923.
2 CW 279, Aug 26, 1923.
3 Solms, cited by Rosky, in Reitz.
4 Freud 1923.
5 Reitz.
6 CW 279, Aug 4, 1922.

6. The Consonants

1 CW 277a, p. 132f.
2 CW 279, July 7, 1924.
3 Kisseleff, CW 277a, p. 59.
4 CW 279, June 24, 1924.
5 CW 282, Sep 21, 1924.
6 CW 218, Oct 22, 1922, and CW 314, Oct 27, 1922.
7 CW 313, April 16, 1921.
8 CW 230, Nov 10, 1923.
9 Glas, MS.
10 CW 170, Aug 15, 1916.
11 Laue 2000.

7. The Vowels

1 CW 279, June 24, 1924.
2 CW 280, p. 67 [Creative Speech, p. 88].
3 CW 305, Aug 24, 1922.
4 CW 267, p. 453, c.1923.
5 Bort p. 52.
6 Barfod 2001.
7 CW 279, June 24, 1924.
8 CW 279, Aug 26, 1923.
9 CW 317, June 30, 1924.
10 July 6, 1924.
11 CW 313, April 12, 1921.
12 CW 27, Chapter 10.
13 Kirchner-Bockholt p. 45.
14 Cosmosophy. Volume 2 (CW 208, Oct 28–30, 1921).

9. The 'Soul Exercises'

1 CW 279, Aug 26, 1923.

10. Transforming Eurythmy

1 CW 279, Aug 26, 1923.
2 CW 277a, p. 22.
3 CW 279, Aug 4, 1922.
4 CW 279, Aug 26, 23.

13. Embryological Gestures

1 Cosmosophy, Volume 2, CW 208, Oct 28, 1921.
2 Laue 2004.
3 Fundamentals of Therapy CW 27, Chapter 5, and LAUE 2000.
4 Cosmosophy, Volume 2, CW 208, Oct 29, 1921.
5 'The Invisible Human Being Within Us,' CW 221, Feb 11, 1923.

14. Therapeutic Words

1 Laue 1999, Laue 2003.
2 Kirchner-Bockholt, Chapter 12.
3 CW 317, June 30, 1924.
4 Kirchner-Bockholt, Chapter 12.
5 CW 312, March 25, 1920.
6 Kirchner-Bockholt, Chapter 12.
7 Kirchner-Bockholt, p. 196.

15. Future Tasks

1 Bentinck.

16. Outline of a Physiology

1 CW 312, March 22, 1920.
2 CW 313, April 17, 1921.

Bibliography

Authors cited in the text and literature for further study

Barfod, W., Seeger, A., van den Akker, G., Jenaro, E., Hogrefe, B. (1992): *Die drei Urphänomene eurythmischer Bewegung.* Verlag am Goetheanum, Switzerland.

Barfod, W. (2001): *I–A–O and the Eurythmy Meditations.* Mercury Press, USA.

Baumann, E. (1955): *Beiträge zum Heileurythmie-Kurs.* Manuscript.

Bentinck, V. (1996): 'Das reduzierende Element in R. Steiners Heileurythmie-Kurs.' In Niederhäuser-de Jaager, et al. (1996).

Bort, J. (1958): *Heileurythmie mit seelenpflege-bedürftigen Kindern.* Natura Verlag, Switzerland.

Bräuner-Gülow, Gisela, and Gülow, Helge (2005): 'Bewegungstherapien im Vergleich. Heileurythmie, Integrative, Konzentrative und Rhythmische Bewegungstherapie. Eine Standortbestimmung.' *Merkurstab*, Vol. 58, No. 6, pp. 458–64.

Deventer-Wolfram, E.v. (1961): 'Erinnerungen und Gedanken über den Weg der Entstehung der Heileurythmie.' *Blätter für Anthroposophie*, Switzerland Vol. 13, No. 10.

Fintelmann, V. (Ed.) 2003: *Onkologie auf anthroposophischer Grundlage.* Verlag Johannes M. Mayer, Germany.

Freud, S. (1990): *The Ego and the Id.* W.W. Norton & Co, USA.

Glas, M. (1987): *Experiences in Remedial Eurythmy.* Temple Lodge Press, UK.

Glöckler, M. (1997): 'Der besondere Auftrag der Heileurythmie in der Heilpädagogik.' In Grimm (1997).

Göbel, T. (1982): *Die Quellen der Kunst.* Verlag am Goetheanum, Switzerland.

Grimm, R. (1997): *Heilende Kräfte in der Bewegung.* Verlag Freies Geistesleben, Germany.

Heusser, P. (Ed.) (1996): *Heileurythmie und Hygienische Eurythmie.* Verlag am Goetheanum, Switzerland.

Heigl, Martin-Ingbert (2006): 'Artemis, Eurythmie, Sprachgestaltung und Philosophie der Freiheit.' *www.widar.de*

Höller, K. (1996): 'Die vier Äther beim heileurythmischen Vokalisieren und Konsonantieren sowie bei den seelischen Übungen.' In: Niederhäuser-de Jaager, et al. (1996).

Jenaro, E. (1999): *Rudolf Steiners eurythmische Lautordnung.* Verlag Freies Geistesleben, Germany.

Kirchner-Bockholt, M. (2004): *Foundations of Curative Eurythmy.* Floris Books, UK.

Kisseleff, T. (1982): *Eurythmie-Arbeit mit Rudolf Steiner.* Verlag die Pforte, Switzerland.

Laue, H. B. von (1999): 'Natur- und geisteswissenschaftliche Aspekte der Tumorentwicklung.' *Merkurstab*, Vol. 52, No. 3, pp. 145–53.

— (2000): 'Die sieben Lebensprozesse, ihre physiologische Verwandlung und die Krebserkrankung.' *Merkurstab*, Vo. 53, No. 5, pp. 305–16.

— (2003): 'Tumorbiologie.' In Fintelmann (2003).

— (2004): 'Kalzium als Substanz und als Prozess im Menschen.' *Merkurstab*, Vol. 57, No. 2, pp. 78–95.

— (2005): 'Die vier Wesensglieder des Menschen und ihre Tätigkeit mit dem Phosphor.' *Merkurstab*, Vol. 58, No. 6, pp. 428–47.
Müller-Wiedemann, H. (1997): 'Über eine allgemeine Wirksamkeit der Heileurythmie.' In Grimm (1997).
Niederhäuser-de Jaager, D., Müller-Wiedemann, S., Höller, K., Herz, L., Bentinck, V., von Heynitz, S., Authenrieth, E.M., Meili, O. (1996): *Heileurythmie und Hygienische Eurythmie*. Verlag am Goetheanum, Switzerland.
Nissen-Schnürer, M. (2001): *Der bewegte Weg zur Gesundheit. Heileurythmie*. Verlag C. Möllmann, Germany.
Parr, Thomas (1993): *Eurythmie, Rudolf Steiners Bühnenkunst*. Verlag am Goetheanum, Switzerland.
Pompino-Marschall, Bernd (2009): *Introduction to Phonetics*. Walter de Gruyter, USA.
Reitz, G., Rosky, T., Schmidts, R., Urspruch, I. (2005): *Heilsame Bewegung. Musik-, Tanz- und Theatertherapie*. Wissenschaftliche Buchgesellschaft, Germany.
Steinke, U. (1998): *Lesebuch Heileurythmie. Aufzeichnungen aus langjähriger Praxis für Patienten, Ärzte*, Therapeuten. Verlag Ch. Möllmann, Germany.
Torriani, R. (2006): 'Die menschliche Konstitution als Ergebnis des Zusammenwirkens von oberem und unterem Menschen.' *Merkurstab*, Vol. 59, No. 1, pp. 31–46.
Wendler, Jürgen, Seidner, Wolfram, Eysholdt, Ulrich (2005): *Lehrbuch der Phoniatrie und Pädaudiologie*. Georg Thieme Verlag, Germany.
Werner, H., Laue, E. E. von, Laue, H. B. von (1995): 'Die Krankheitsbiographie als diagnostisches und therapeutisches Element.' *Merkurstab*, Vol. 48, No. 2, pp. 177–92.
Wolff-Hoffmann, G. (1986) 'Heileurythmie.' In *Das Bild des Menschen als Grundlage der Heilkunst*. Vol. 2, Verlag Freies Geistesleben, Germany.

Rudolf Steiner

Volumes of the Complete Works (CW) of the works of Rudolf Steiner quoted in the text.
27 *Extending Practical Medicine, Fundamental Principles Based on the Science of the Spirit*, Rudolf Steiner Press 1996.
45 *Anthroposophy (A Fragment)*, SB 2006.
170 *The Riddle of Humanity*, Rudolf Steiner Press 1990.
208 *Cosmosophy*, Vol. 2: *Cosmic Influences on the Human Being*, Completion Press
221 *Earthly Knowledge and Heavenly Wisdom*, Anthroposophic Press 1991.
230 *Harmony of the Creative World*, (previously *Man as Symphony of the Creative Word*), Rudolf Steiner Press 2001.
267 *Seelenübungen*, Vol. 1 [Soul Exercises, not translated] Rudolf Steiner Verlag, Switzerland 2001.
277a *Eurythmy: Its Birth and Development*, Anastasi 2002.
279 *Eurythmy as Visible Speech*, Rudolf Steiner Press 1984.
280 *Creative Speech*, Rudolf Steiner Press 1999.
282 *Speech and Drama*, SB 2007
300b *Faculty Meetings with Rudolf Steiner*, Vol. 1, Anthroposophic Press 1998.
303 *Soul Economy*, SB 2003.
305 *The Spiritual Ground of Education*, SB 2004.
312 *Introducing Anthroposophical Medicine*, SB 2010.
313 *Anthroposophical Spiritual Science and Medical Therapy*, Mercury Press 1991.
314 In three different volumes: *Physiology and Therapeutics*, Mercury Press 1986. *Fundamentals of Anthroposophical Medicine*, Mercury Press 1986. ; *Health Care as a Social Issue*, Mercury Press 1984.
315 *Eurythmy Therapy*, Rudolf Steiner Press 2009.
317 *Education for Special Needs: The Curative Education Course*, Rudolf Steiner Press 1998.

Index

You may also be interested in

Anthroposophical Care for the Elderly
Annegret Camps, Brigitte Hagenhoff and Ada van der Star

Anthroposophical Therapeutic Speech
Barbara Denjean-von Stryk and Dietrich von Bonin

Biographical Work: The Anthroposophical Basis
Gudrun Burkhard

*Compresses and other Therapeutic Applications:
A Handbook from the Ita Wegman Clinic*
Monika Fingado

Foundations of Anthroposophical Medicine: A Training Manual
Edited by Guus van der Bie and Machteld Huber

Foundations of Curative Eurythmy
Margarete Kirchner-Bockholt

Rhythmic Einreibung: A Handbook from the Ita Wegman Clinic
Monika Fingado

The Background to Anthroposophical Therapeutic Speech
Edited by Dietrich von Bonin

Foundations of Curative Eurythmy

Margarete Kirchner-Bockholt

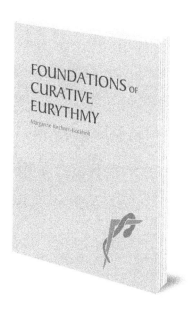

In 1921 Rudolf Steiner gave a series of lectures on curative eurythmy. Over the subsequent years, as advice was sought in particular cases of illness, he added to the initial exercises and indications. For the benefit of those who did not attend the original courses, Dr Kirchner-Bockholt published the basic principles, along with an authentic collection of Steiner's advice.

This is Dr Kirchner-Bockholt's comprehensive handbook. It is both a guide for curative eurythmists in their work, and an introduction to the therapy for the general practitioner.

www.florisbooks.co.uk

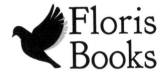
Floris Books

For news on all our **latest books**,
and to receive **exclusive discounts**,
join our mailing list at:

florisbooks.co.uk

Plus subscribers get a FREE book
with every online order!

Printed in the USA
CPSIA information can be obtained
at www.ICGtesting.com
JSHW011519221024
72172JS00009B/77